KNOW THYSELF

Yoga Philosophy Made Accessible

Gudjon Bergmann

Table of Contents

FOREWORD 7

THE POPULARITY OF YOGA 9

MY BACKGROUND IN YOGA 10

MAKING YOGA ACCESSIBLE...................................11

YOGA: A PATH TO SELF-REALIZATION 13

THE BODY, MIND AND SPIRIT 13

HOW WELL DO YOU KNOW YOUR SELF? 15

PRECIOUS FEW SEARCH FOR THE TRUTH....................16

THE UPSIDE OF YOGA PRACTICE............................17

YOGA IS A VEHICLE FOR SELF-EXPLORATION 18

SCIENTIFIC EXPLORATION....................................18

ELEMENT OF FAITH...19

ATMAN – THE ETERNAL SELF.................................20

WHEN THE STUDENT IS READY 23

OBSERVANCES FOR YOGA STUDENTS...........................24

STAIN ON A WHITE PIECE OF CLOTH 27

TO CONSIDER WHEN CHOOSING A TEACHER............. 29

... THE TEACHER WILL APPEAR 30

THE MAIN PATHS OF YOGA 31

THE GOAL OF YOGA PRACTICE 33

AN INTEGRAL OR HOLISTIC APPROACH....................... 34

GNANA YOGA 37

THE GNANA YOGA PRAYER.. 39

MAYA – THE COSMIC ILLUSION.................................... 39

TO READ BEFORE AND AFTER MEDITATION............... 42

KARMA YOGA 45

DIFFERENT KINDS OF REACTION 46

KARMA YOGA AND REINCARNATION........................... 47

SWA-DHARMA = PERSONAL PATH................................ 50

BHAKTI YOGA 53

VIVEKANANDA ON 9/11/1893...................................... 53

THE MANY FACES OF GOD 56

BRAHMAN.. 56

ISHWARA = GOD 57

POLYTHEISM OR MONOTHEISM 57

NADA YOGA 58

EVERYONE CAN PRAY 60

TRUE WORSHIP 61

CHRISTIAN CONNECTION 62

PATH OF LOVE AND COMPASSION 62

RAJA YOGA (ASHTANGA) 65

DELVING DEEPER 70

1. YAMA (SELF-CONTROL) 70

2. NIYAMA (POSITIVE ATTRIBUTES)............74

3. ASANA (POSTURE) 77

4. PRANAYAMA (ENERGY CONTROL)...........78

5. PRATYAHARA (SENSE CONTROL)..............79

6. DHARANA (CONCENTRATION) 81

7. DHYANA (MEDITATION) 83

8. SAMADHI (SELF-REALIZATION) 85

HATHA YOGA (KUNDALINI) 87

HEALTH BENEFITS... 87

SEVEN CATEGORIES... 88

CONTROLLING LIFE ENERGY... 91

KUNDALINI WARNINGS.. 93

HATHA YOGA IS SAFE... 94

EPILOGUE ON RAJA/HATHA YOGA......................... 95

REGULAR PRACTICE.. 97

TEMPORARY STATES – PERMANENT TRAITS............... 97

RAJA AND HATHA YOGA PRACTICE............................... 98

KARMA YOGA PRACTICE.. 99

BHAKTI YOGA PRACTICE... 100

GNANA YOGA PRACTICE.. 100

HOLISTIC OR INTEGRAL PRACTICE............................. 101

DANGERS ON THE SPIRITUAL PATH.................... 103

THE DARTH VADER SYNDROME.................................... 103

ESCAPISM... 104

CO-DEPENDENCY... 105

VANITY... 105

EXTERNAL NORMS.. 106

ETHICAL DETERIORATION 107

LAZINESS 107

LACK OF PATIENCE AND PERSISTENCE 108

IN YOUR HANDS 111

APPENDIX 1 SANSKRIT GLOSSARY 113

APPENDIX 2 RECOMMENDED READING 123

APPENDIX 3 GUDJON BERGMANN'S

BIBLIOGRAPHY 125

Yes! You Can Manage Stress (2011) 125

Motivation & Peace of Mind (2011) 125

Quit Smoking and Be Free! (2011) 125

Balance: The Seven Human Needs Simplified (2011) ... 126

Create a Safe Space (2011) 126

Living in the Spirit of Yoga (2010) 127

The Seven Human Needs (2006) 128

Books in Icelandic - Out of Print 129

FOREWORD

Gudjon Bergmann is a skilled educator, scholar, writer and lecturer. It is the result of his relentless search and dedication for truth during his entire life. He has fundamental qualities required for the search. He has intense desire for learning, dedication, enthusiasm, questioning, exploring and making sacrifices for the truth. He is well read in Western philosophy and psychology and has explored Eastern mysticism in a scientific way. He has traveled extensively to reach the real source of wisdom by meeting original revolutionary masters. He has blended Eastern and Western philosophies in a concise and practical way.

Gudjon has studied with me personally for the last fourteen years. He has visited me frequently and I have stayed with his family during our teacher training sessions in Iceland. These encounters have given him the depth and understanding of the practical application of yoga in daily life. We have communicated constantly over the years. He has asked sincere questions, which is required for exploration of truth, and has deep humility to receive the wisdom.

I have relied on his expertise and experience to edit and organize my publications.

In this book he gives clear understanding of four major paths of self-realization. He goes in details about *Raja Yoga* and *Hatha Yoga* practices. He gives practical application to integrate practices in life. He has clearly pointed out the fads, dilutions and distortions in the name of yoga. He also describes aids and obstacles on the spiritual path.

This book is the eye opener for all who want to explore yoga in a capsule form. It is a great guide for yoga teachers who hold certificates and teach only physical yoga. They will benefit from this book to enrich their practice and teaching, and will be able to provide greater service to their students.

Yogi Shanti Desai
www.yogishantidesai.com

THE POPULARITY OF YOGA

In the last thirty to forty years, practices related to yoga have become increasingly popular in the West, especially practices that have to do with physical exercises. This popularity has achieved two polar opposites. At one end it has increased the exposure of yoga and at the other end it has diluted the real essence of yoga. The dilution is very visible. In some cases the term yoga has become a fashionable marketing term and has been intertwined with all kinds of products and exercises previously unrelated to yoga. The positive aspect is that more people are now open to the ideas presented by yoga philosophy than ever before. The goal of this book is to make the philosophy of yoga accessible to everyone who is interested in learning more.

The deepest understanding of yoga will never appeal to everyone. In fact, some aspects of yoga are so specialized that they can only be practiced by those who have cast aside their worldly attachments and decided to invest all their waking hours in the practice and fulfillment of yoga. On the other hand there are many ideas in yoga philosophy and many yogic practices that most everyone can benefit from learning and applying in their life. In this book it is my intention to emphasize the core concepts of yoga. My goal is to make yoga philosophy accessible and I intend to use simple everyday language along with traditional *Sanskrit* terminology to achieve that goal.

To begin with I will describe the purpose of yoga practice. Next I will explain the observances that a student of yoga must develop to gain traction in his practice. Then I will clarify the main branches of yoga philosophy and the different paths that are available to all of us. After that I will show how the philosophy transforms into practices and will set the stage for an integral or holistic yoga practice. Near the end you will find a *Sanskrit* glossary of the main yoga concepts, a list of relevant books for in depth reading, and my bibliography.

MY BACKGROUND IN YOGA

I am a yoga educator, a pundit so to speak, and have been a student and practitioner of yoga since early 1997. Earlier in my life I was introduced to a variety of spiritual practices, but within yoga I discovered a holistic approach that resonated with me at a deep level.

In 1998 I graduated from a yoga teacher training administered by Asmundur Gunnlaugsson and Yogi Shanti Desai in my native country of Iceland. Through the years, Yogi Shanti Desai, who is a Western minded disciple of Swami Kripalu, has become my mentor and friend.

I ran my own yoga studio in Iceland from 2001 to 2006 and have taught yoga postures for well over 6000 hours. I have also trained 80 yoga teachers, written and published a number of books on yoga, taught yoga on TV, written dozens of articles about yoga, published a yoga DVD, and published a number of relaxation CD's.

In 2004 I attended a 500 hour advanced teacher training with Sri Yogi Hari, a direct disciple of Swami Vishnu-Devananda, the man responsible for opening Sivananda Yoga Centers all over the world. At his ashram in Florida I learned *Sampoorna Yoga* and deepened my understanding of yoga philosophy and learned the essence of mantra chanting or *Nada Yoga*.

I have kept up my practice over the years and repeatedly read and studied all the major texts of yoga. I had a very powerful spiritual awakening at the age of eighteen, years, before I was introduced to yoga, but I have by no means reached the permanent state of enlightenment, even though I pass into the meditative state with more ease now than I ever did before. When writing this book I put trust in my teachers and in the original texts of yoga.

MAKING YOGA ACCESSIBLE

As a yoga educator I have always focused on making yoga accessible to the public by teaching the practical aspects of yoga. This book presents a vital part of that process, as do my previous books in English, especially *Living in the Spirit of Yoga* (2010) and *Create a Safe Space* (2010). The reader does not need to agree with all the philosophies of yoga to benefit from reading this book. I have done my best to present and interpret the major paths of yoga, but even I do not subscribe to all the mythic beliefs portrayed in yoga philosophy. I do believe that the core philosophies reveal an important reality, a part of life often overlooked by scientific Western minds, and I firmly believe in the core concepts of yoga, otherwise I would not be a practitioner. Please feel free to approach this book like a buffet. If you don't like something, simply skip over it and enjoy other parts that are more palatable to you at the moment. Who knows, your appetite may change.

Gudjon Bergmann
www.gudjonbergmann.com

YOGA: A PATH TO SELF-REALIZATION

The goal of yoga is to attain harmony between body and mind and fully realize the ever present spirit, thus attaining unity between body, mind and spirit. Yoga can be presented as a *philosophy*, a *practice*, a *state of being*, or all of the above. The *philosophy* of yoga contains ideas about man's purpose on this Earth. The *practices* of yoga give people the tools for self-realization, and if pursued they will lead us to the *state* of yoga, which is also known as *samadhi* or enlightenment, the first-hand account and experience of the spirit, known as *Atman* in yoga philosophy. According to yoga, temporary heightened states or religious experiences can be reached by a variety of means, but only through a systematic practice (see chapter on *Raja Yoga*) can temporary states be turned into permanent traits.

THE BODY, MIND AND SPIRIT

The body, mind and spirit are reflected in three *states* that everyone goes through over a period of twenty four hours, namely waking, dreaming, and deep sleep. According to yoga philosophy the *material realm* or body is represented by the waking state, the *astral realm* or thought is represented by the dreaming state, and the *causal realm* or spirit is represented by deep dreamless sleep.

When you are in the waking state, you are aware of the body and everything that is related to the body, but as soon as you fall asleep, your body might as well not exist. You leave the material realm and enter the astral realm. When dreaming, the mind can conjure up all kinds of images and ideas, good and bad, all the while sifting through the information and experiences you have encountered while waking. But even though you are not aware of your body while dreaming, you still have a sense of identity; you are still you, even though the mental image you conjure up in your mind may be different from your physical appearance. When dreaming subsides, and this happens intermittently during the night, you enter into deep dreamless sleep. Few things are known about this state, other than it seems to be vital to the mental and physical health of human beings. In deep dreamless sleep you get a deep peaceful rest and go through a rejuvenation process without which your body could not exist. But even though you are not thinking in the state of deep sleep, there is still an identity, there is still consciousness.

One of the ailments in modern society is lack of deep dreamless sleep. Such a lack can induce tiredness, physical pain and mental irritation, such as anxiety and harmful stress. With the constant intake of information, the mind needs more 'computing' time during sleep, i.e. more dreaming, and that can result in less deep dreamless sleep. The practices of yoga can be very helpful in that regard, regulating waking and sleeping rhythms.

HOW WELL DO YOU KNOW YOUR SELF?

Thinking about these three distinctly different states that you go through *every 24 hours*, you can begin to answer an interesting question. How much self-knowledge have you actually accumulated through the years?

Let us first examine the waking state. Very few people know their body well enough, even while waking. If more people would listen to the natural rhythms of the body and *rest* when tired, *exercise* when restless, *eat* when hungry and *stop eating* when full, we would be dealing with fewer diseases overall and people would have more energy.

What about the mental state represented by dreaming; the realm of thought? In my line of work as a yoga teacher and stress management consultant, I have found that people in general have very little control over their thoughts. It is much easier to control the body than it is to control the mind, simply because the body is measureable and people only use a fraction of the mind to control it. Through the ages many people have set out to map the mind and we still don't have a conclusive map. Having said that, yogis, mystics and modern scientists have all made contributions to illuminate thought processes and society has benefitted greatly from their endeavors. But we can expect that much time will pass before the mapping of the mind is complete. Thus it can be said that no one knows the entirety of their mind.

To be fair, most people know their body and mind to a degree, but when it comes to defining or discussing the causal state, which is related to deep dreamless sleep, most people find themselves stumped. What happens in deep dreamless sleep? It's hard to tell. Consciousness and identity are still there, but consciousness is not thinking and does not sense the body.

PRECIOUS FEW SEARCH FOR THE TRUTH

Performing this short and very simple mental exercise usually has people feeling that they don't know themselves very well at all. You may ask: "Do I really need more self-knowledge?" It's a good and worthy question. There are a million other things competing for your attention in life. Why spend precious time on treading the arduous and time consuming path of self-discovery?

Sufficient to say, this is not a new dilemma. In the ancient text *Bhagavad-Gita*, Krishna says that out of thousands only *one* searches for the truth. Krishna then proceeds to say that out of a thousand men searching only *one* will find the truth.

THE UPSIDE OF YOGA PRACTICE

Even if complete self-knowledge is *not* your end goal, minimal efforts in the direction of self-knowledge can yield some *very positive results*, such as:

- Increased *physical awareness,* which can result in better overall health and wellbeing, especially with the aid of yoga postures, which have become very popular in the West
- Increased awareness and control over the *thought-waves in the mind* will result in mental and emotional stability
- And if you open yourself up to the concept of *Atman,* the soul, the self, the unchanging witness or spirit (whatever you want to call that which is beyond the realm of names), you can experience more moments of calm, serenity and peace of mind

Increased self-knowledge yields real and practical results that everyone can benefit from, even if they don't reach the ultimate goal described in the ancient yogic texts.

YOGA IS A VEHICLE FOR SELF-EXPLORATION

The second yoga sutra says: "*Yoga is the control of thought-waves in the mind*" (in *Sanskrit* it is *Yogas Chitta Vritti Nirodaha*), also translated as the *calming* of the thought-waves. By gaining more control over the thought-waves each man, woman and child has the possibility of experiencing *turiya*, the fourth state of consciousness, which has been likened to *conscious or wakeful deep dreamless sleep*. The goal of yoga is to tame the mind and body so that a direct perception of the spirit or *Atman* (which is always present in states of waking, dreaming and deep dreamless sleep even though we are not always aware of this unchanging reality behind the scenes) can occur.

The spirit or *Atman* has three distinct qualities according to yoga philosophy. They are *Sat* (absolute truth), *Chit* (absolute knowledge) and *Anand* (absolute bliss). The supreme goal of yoga is enlightenment (*samadhi*), being constantly connected to the source of life, the unchanging *Atman*. That is purpose of yoga in a nutshell.

SCIENTIFIC EXPLORATION

No outside sources can confirm or deny the existence of *Atman*, but a scientific exploration can be performed through *personal practice*. The ancient yogis developed a scientific approach which was rather simple. A group of practicing yogis would meet and compare notes about their meditative experiences. In his book *The Marriage of Sense and Soul*, philosopher Ken Wilber, which has greatly influenced my work, describes how the scientific methods used in mathematics and psychology can be used in the area of spiritual exploration, essentially through *practice* and *comparison*. Only practicing mathematicians can partake in a comparison when dealing with mathematics, and the same is true in relation to yoga practices. Only the practitioners can compare, based on the knowledge and experiences they have derived from their practice. In the case of yoga, a body of work was born over a long period of time, and that work was eventually written down. This process of practice and comparison produced most of the yoga scriptures. But the problem with writing anything down is that it tends to slow down evolution, since words on paper are often taken quite literally. We must keep that in mind when contemplating the future evolution of yoga.

ELEMENT OF FAITH

If the yoga practitioner decides to invest time and energy in his yoga practice, he is operating on an *element of faith* even though his practice may be scientific. He must trust that those who came before him are speaking truthfully. The yoga practitioner is *not required* to believe anything, rather, he is urged to *practice* and *experience*.

19

The practice of yoga is the scientific endeavor of travelling consciously deep into the mind, beyond thoughts, words and concepts, and unravel the mysteries of the deep dreamless state. Whether this will become standard psychology in the future or remain a spiritual process is yet to be determined, but it is a vital part in the process of gathering self-knowledge.

ATMAN – THE ETERNAL SELF

According to yoga philosophy, the spirit, or *Atman*, is an *ever present* silent witness or pure consciousness. In order to experience *Atman* directly, one must unlearn much of the conditioning that *Maya*, which is the *ever changing* material world of light and shadows, has imprinted upon the human psyche. In addition to obvious yoga practices, unlearning and discernment are a big part of yoga practice and philosophy.

The concept of *Atman* has deep reaching implications. The following verse, which is taken from the *Bhagavad-Gita*, describes *Atman*. It is my personal favorite and has been a source of inspiration and guided me through some tough times.

When my father died in 2004 I read this verse over and over again to my considerable consolation. My father had a similar saying. He never understood the purpose of visiting a graveyard, and often said: *"You would never go to a car-cemetery to visit the driver."*

Know this Atman
Unborn, undying,
Never ceasing,
Never beginning,
Deathless, birthless,
Unchanging forever.
How can It die
The death of the body?

Knowing It birthless,
Knowing It deathless,
Knowing It endless,
Forever unchanging,
Dream not you do
The deed of the killer,
Dream not the power
Is yours to command it.

Worn-out garments
Are shed by the body:
Worn-out bodies
Are shed by the dweller
Within the body.
New bodies are donned

By the dweller, like garments.

Not wounded by weapons,
Not burned by fire,
Not dried by the wind,
Not wetted by water:
Such is the Atman,
Not dried, not wetted,
Not burned, not wounded,
Innermost element,
Everywhere, always,
Being of beings,
Changeless, eternal,
Forever and ever.

Verse from the *Bhagavad-Gita: The Song of God* translated by Swami Prabhavananda & Christopher Isherwood.

I encourage you to read this verse often, meditate on its meaning, and explore within, to see if you can confirm the existence of *Atman* or spirit in your own life.

WHEN THE STUDENT IS READY ...

I have long contemplated the phrase "*When the student is ready, the teacher will appear*" and the actual meaning becomes ever clearer in my mind. The process of learning is not only based on a teacher's ability to teach, but also on a students' ability to receive. People who have been in the presence of master teachers have often overlooked the wisdom of their teachings because they were not open and receptive. This becomes doubly important when applied to spiritual teachings. For a long time I misinterpreted the phrase and thought that when I would be ready I would find *one teacher* or *guru* that would teach me everything I needed to know. I was looking for the one person who would lead me out of the darkness. That is actually what the term *guru* means, *gu* means darkness and *ru* means light. The *guru* leads the student from the darkness of material bondage to the light of spiritual life. I was so busy waiting for the one *guru*, that I overlooked many of the teachers I was meeting along the way. For example, it took me a while to really appreciate the teachings and guidance of Yogi Shanti Desai, but every time I met him, my respect for him grew. As I uncovered my lack of knowledge I became more humble. *Humility* and *respect* are key aspects in the process of learning. When I met Sri Yogi Hari in Florida in 2004 I was better prepared, as I had already been learning with Yogi Shanti Desai for almost six years. From the time I entered his *ashram* I did my best to be humble and respectful, although I freely admit that it wasn't always easy. My approach worked and I walked away from the five hundred hour advanced yoga teacher training much the wiser. But humility and respect are not the only ingredients a yoga practitioner needs in order to become a good student.

OBSERVANCES FOR YOGA STUDENTS

According to yoga philosophy, a true student of yoga should cultivate the following five observances if he wants to amplify his yoga practice and adhere to yogic wisdom. These observances are meant as guidelines. Aim for progress instead of perfection.

1. *Mumuksha* (desire for enlightenment). A yoga practitioner should cultivate a desire for increased self-knowledge and enlightenment. A person that wants to commit to a physical exercise program must first discover a desire for exercise. If the person has no desire, or if the desire isn't strong enough, then the person will not be willing to persist through the inevitable difficulties associated with starting a physical exercise routine.

The same thing can be said about anyone who wants to train the mind. A person wanting to train the mind must have encountered mental irritation and discomfort, or found other motivating reasons, in order for her to persist through the process of making mental changes (which by the way is a lot more difficult than starting an exercise program).

In order for a person to act on spiritual teachings and maintain *years* of meditation practice and other observances, the desire for *samadhi* or enlightenment must be strong. In fact the student must be fed up with many of the worldly desires he has pursued to no avail.

2. *Viveka* (discernment). Being able to discern between beneficial and unhelpful practices is a very important observance. The yoga practitioner should cultivate the ability to discern the real from the unreal, discern between permanent and impermanent states, and discern between truth and lies. He must cultivate discernment to choose a path that will in the end lead to *samadhi*, to freedom – because in the process he must trust others who have tread the path before him and there is no shortage of spiritual "snake-oil salesmen" in this world.

3. Vairagya (non-attachment). A strong mind and the bravery to relinquish attachment to worldly objects are two things that should be at the heart of a yoga practitioner's life. When the practitioner realizes that *Maya*, the world of illusions, eventually leads to both mental and physical suffering, he begins to observe non-attachment to the ever changing nature of the world. This does not mean that he practices apathy; simply that he is aware of the changing nature of *Maya* and seeks to strengthen his bond to the constant and unchanging reality, *Atman*. Non-attachment to an ever changing world will eventually lead to enlightenment, while apathy and disinterest will not.

4. Abhyasa (constant practice). Constant practice is the result of a strong desire for enlightenment, discernment and non-attachment. No one can reap benefits without sowing seeds. The yoga practitioner sows by ardently practicing all that he has been taught.

5. Satsang (gathering of truth). To make sure that he doesn't regress back to his old ways of living, the yoga practitioner surrounds himself with mentors, teachers and fellow students who are on the spiritual path. He reads spiritual books and surrounds himself with constructive and supportive energy. The word *sangha* means gathering and the word *sat* means truth. Thus *Satsang* is literally the gathering of truth.

STAIN ON A WHITE PIECE OF CLOTH

It's good to realize from the beginning that no teacher is perfect. *Being human is the same as being imperfect.* I have been fortunate enough to interact with many spiritually inclined individuals over the years, and developed a relationship with a few select spiritually evolved teachers; people who have proactively sought personal and spiritual growth through various means. These people have taught me so much that my lifespan will hardly suffice to put it all into practice. But one of the most important lessons I have learned has not come from their books or lectures, but from my interactions with them. The metaphor that best describes this important lesson is *"a stain on a white piece of cloth"*. Let me explain.

People who are involved in personal and spiritual growth, even those who are called spiritual masters, can still display damaging personality flaws. You only need to observe Howard Gardner's multiple intelligence theory to see mismatches between aptitudes. But because these people are so exemplary in the spiritual arena, their flaws become about as apparent as stains become on a white piece of cloth. I have often had to dig deep in order to look past flaws and benefit from very important knowledge that my teachers have imparted.

Many personal development and spiritual teachers get attacked by their peers for the few stains that are left on their otherwise white piece of cloth and little praise for all the good they have done. These attacks are usually based on unrealistic expectations.

The other side of the coin is also worth noting. White spots can become very visible on an otherwise dirty cloth. Sometimes extremely flawed people get praise for uncharacteristic acts of kindness, because it contrasts with their otherwise rude demeanor.

By presenting this metaphor I am in *no way encouraging people to look past flaws* that they may perceive when they interact with spiritual teachers. I am simply asking you, the reader, not to overlook all the good you can potentially learn from a person simply because you spot an apparent stain or character flaw. The best teachers are often wounded healers. Men and women who have overcome difficulty in their lives, learned from them, and can therefore teach others, both by sharing spiritual nuggets of gold and by recounting their experiences.

TO CONSIDER WHEN CHOOSING A TEACHER

When choosing a spiritual teacher, guide or mentor, it's good to have the following three guidelines in mind. Their teachings should be in line with:

1. *Common Sense* – Whatever the teacher is saying should not go against everything that you have ever been taught. Truth is universal. Use common sense to identify impostors. And don't choose a *guru* or teacher that is either dead or inaccessible. You need a guide that is available and can teach you personally.

2. *The Original Scriptures* – If you are in doubt about what is being taught and don't think it corresponds with the original scriptures (although scriptures always need to be interpreted, I am not encouraging literal thinking), then you can always consult original texts such as the *Bhagavad-Gita*, the *Upanishads* or Patanjalis *Yoga Sutras*. If the teachings are far removed from the original texts, then you are not likely to be getting the guidance you are seeking.

3. *The Lives of the Masters* – Examine the lives of spiritual masters such as Gandhi, Paramahansa Yogananda, Ramakrishna, Vivekananda, and Mother Teresa, or the current life of someone like the Dalai Lama. Do the teachings you

are receiving rhyme with what you see reflected in the lives of the masters? Also look into the life of the teacher you are studying with. Does he adhere to his own theories and practices most of the time?

... THE TEACHER WILL APPEAR

According to yoga philosophy man is blessed with free will and the ability to doubt and discern. These abilities will lead him to teachers, guides and mentors that can give him guidance on the path towards self-discovery. Cultivate the attitudes and observances of a true student and you will meet teachers wherever you look, because *learning is in the mind of the student.*

THE MAIN PATHS OF YOGA

Many people become confused about the seemingly many paths being offered when they start practicing yoga, but at the core there are only *four main paths of yoga*, and they have the same end goal which is *samadhi* or enlightenment. The end goal can be likened to the top of a pyramid. Even though people may start climbing the pyramid from different sides, at the end they will reach the same goal and thusly achieve unity.

In yoga philosophy people's personality types are divided into three main groups. One group is driven by *action*, the second group is driven by *emotion* and the third group is driven by *intellect*. Even though personalities are thusly divided it doesn't mean that a person that is mainly driven by emotion neither thinks nor acts. Everyone has access to all three traits, but usually one is dominant. The four main paths of yoga revolve around these groups or categories. Depending upon which personality trait is dominant, you can choose a yoga practice to fit your tendencies.

- A person that is driven by action practices *Karma Yoga*, the path of action, or *Raja Yoga*, the path of scientific practice
- A person that is driven by emotion practices *Bhakti Yoga*, the path of love and devotion
- A person that is driven by intellect practices *Gnana Yoga*, the path of intellectual discernment and contemplation

Within the diverse world of yoga you can find other paths, but they all fall under one of these four major categories. For example, the popular physical aspect of yoga, called *Hatha Yoga*, which includes postures and energy manipulation, falls under the practice of *Raja Yoga*. Within the *Hatha Yoga* category, you will find a variety of newly formed *brands* or *trademarks* that have entered the market in the past few decades, including *Iyengar*, *Bikram*, *Anusara*, *Astanga*, *Kripalu* and more (see glossary for details). These are all branded variations of *Hatha Yoga*, and are the main cause for people's confusion about the perceived variety within yoga.

As mentioned earlier, the popularity of yoga has made it a sought after marketing concept and we are now at the point where many people have interjected the word yoga in their brand even though their practices are far removed from the philosophies and core practices of yoga. This trend is likely to continue, which increases the need for thoughtful discernment.

THE GOAL OF YOGA PRACTICE

According to yoga philosophy, body, mind and spirit are also called the *material body*, the *astral body* and the *causal body*. These are the bodies of consciousness.

When you are dreaming you are not conscious of your material body, it might as well not exist at that point because consciousness travels within the astral realm, the realm of thoughts, concepts and images. When you enter the state of deep dreamless sleep, you lose conscious awareness of your thoughts. The astral body is thusly discarded the same way the material body was before it and all that remains is the causal body.

According to yoga philosophy the causal body is *Atman*, our deepest core. It has the qualities of absolute truth (*sat*), absolute knowledge or wisdom (*chit*) and absolute bliss (*anand*). However, most people have no conscious recollection of entering this state when they awake after a good night's sleep. The goal of yoga practice is to make the practitioner aware of the causal body, through the practice of drawing attention away from the material and astral bodies; *consciously entering the state of deep dreamless sleep is* therefore called *turyia* or the fourth state, which is also known as the meditative state. *Everything that follows in this book is based on this core understanding of yoga.*

AN INTEGRAL OR HOLISTIC APPROACH

Even though the original scriptures divide yoga into four paths, my teachers and main influencers have emphasized an integral or holistic approach. They suggest that the student should combine practices from all the major paths, sort of like *spiritual cross training.*

Yogi Shanti Desai published the *Yoga Holistic Practice Manual* many years ago and as the title suggest he emphasizes a holistic approach.

Sri Yogi Hari has a *Sanskrit* name for his approach and calls it *Sampoorna Yoga,* which simply means full, complete or whole. It is a combination of *Raja, Gnana, Bhakti* and *Karma* Yoga. He also emphasizes *Hatha Yoga* (physical postures which fall under the path of *Raja*) and *Nada Yoga* (the yoga of vibration which includes mantra chanting and falls under the path of *Bhakti*).

Both teachers emphasize a whole, complete or integral approach that can be likened to a bird. The head represents *Gnana Yoga,* the intellect and discernment that guides the bird. The wings are *Bhakti* and *Karma Yoga,* the bird uses actions and devotion to propel himself. The tail is *Raja Yoga,* which the bird uses to direct his energies.

In the following chapters the four main paths of yoga will be explained in more detail.

GNANA YOGA

The word *Gnana* means wisdom or knowledge (to avoid confusion I must point out that the word is sometimes spelled with a J as *Jnana*). *Gnana Yoga* is the path of self-discovery and self-knowledge. Yoga philosophy claims that the highest goal is to know ones core, the Self, the Witness, the Spirit, *Atman*. It is said that worldly knowledge is represented with the number *zero*, while self-knowledge is represented with the number *one*. Only when worldly knowledge (0) is preceded with self-knowledge (1) does worldly knowledge become valuable (10).

Gnana Yoga is a perfect path for intellectual people who are swayed towards logic. *It is the philosopher's yoga.* The practitioner of *Gnana Yoga* uses his own mind as a laboratory. His main goal is to peer beyond the unreal to discover everlasting truth. He uses the words *Neti, Neti* (not this, not that) to dive deep into the nature of his own existence.

The first assumption of *Gnana Yoga* is that for *Ultimate Reality* to be ultimately real, it has to be *permanent*. If it changes, then it is not ultimate reality, merely relative reality. The practitioner of *Gnana Yoga* is attempting uncover the layers of his own core and expose the part of him that was never born and will never die.

Modern physics show us very clearly that material is never destroyed only *transformed*. At its core all material is energy and at the core of energy is consciousness. When you burn a stick you are not destroying the stick, only transforming it into ashes and air particles. What then is at the core of the stick? Is it wood, heat, air, ashes, energy, consciousness, or something else?

With a simple exploration of the world around us we quickly find that not everything is as it seems. Our senses often deceive us. From our standpoint we see a rug. When the rug is put under a microscope we discover a forest full of organisms. If we peer deeper we find pure energy. Being sensible (using the five senses to perceive and analyze the surrounding world) is therefore a very limited way of exploring the permanent or unchanging nature of things.

What is real in the world? What is the underlying core that never changes even though matter is constantly being transformed? The goal of *Gnana Yoga* is to uncover this core through introspection using questions such as: Who am I? What is the nature of my mind? Where did I come from? What is the purpose of my life? What is the purpose of human existence? What happens after death? What is ultimately real and permanent?

THE GNANA YOGA PRAYER

Asatoma Sadgamaya
Lead me from the unreal to the real
Tamasoma Jyotirgamaya
Lead me from the darkness of ignorance
to the light of knowledge
Mrityorma Amritamgamaya
Lead me from the fear of death to
the acknowledgement of immortality

MAYA – THE COSMIC ILLUSION

What prevents the *Gnana Yoga* practitioner from knowing his core instantly? According to yoga philosophy it is the seductive power of the material world, also known as *Maya*. Long before Albert Einstein theorized about the nature of the universe, the ancient *rishis* (seers) discovered that the world is really a mirage, a play of lights and shadows. Today's physicists use similar verbiage to describe the world. The material that we perceive to be solid is really pure energy or 99.9999% emptiness. From a *limited, time bound standpoint*, the material world is real; from a *permanent or absolute standpoint*, the names, forms and definitions we attach ourselves to daily are a mirage and ultimately unreal.

According to yoga philosophy the seductive power of this play of lights and shadows hides the underlying truth from us. Our senses deceive us every waking moment. Everything that we can see, touch, hear, smell or taste, is bound to the impermanent constrains of time and space. *Gnana Yoga* focuses on peering through these mirages and discovering permanence or ultimate reality.

At first glance *Gnana Yoga* may appear to be simple and easy, but it takes courage and discipline to constantly face the deceptions that the mind and body perceive as true. Peering into ultimate reality may lead to desperation and indifference. If everything is unreal, if the world is an illusion, then what is the point in living?

Gnana Yoga is not about denying relative material reality. All practitioners must adhere to relative natural laws, such as going to the toilet, sleeping, eating, etc. The point is simply to peer deeper and become aware of the underlying ultimate reality. That is why it is good for the *Gnana Yoga* practitioner to have a teacher or spiritual guide who has already travelled along this path. It is also wise to use the *synergy* of a holistic yoga practice. The love of *Bhakti Yoga*, the action and work of *Karma Yoga* and the discipline of *Raja Yoga* can ease the struggle when the practitioner is peering through mirages to discover ultimate reality.

An old yogic metaphor likens it to turning on the light in a darkened room where the shape of a rope has produced the mirage of a snake and caused fear. Once the light has been turned on, even if it is only for a moment, the fear of the imagined snake simply disappears.

When the *Gnana Yoga* practitioner sees himself and the world clearly, it is like he awakens from a dream and finds himself to be an actor on stage in a play called life. At that point he is faced with a choice. Does he keep on acting, now aware of his real identity, or does the discovery cause him such anguish that he sits down and stops acting?

Many people have used the discovery of *Maya*, the world of illusion, to turn away from life and stop playing their roles. But *Karma Yoga* reminds us to stick to our roles, to keep working without attachment, to adhere to our duty, and be ever mindful of the fact that we are simply playing a role. The role of a parent is to look after his offspring, the role of a spouse is to support his mate, the role of a child is to play and learn, the role of an employee is to work, the role of a teacher is to teach and so on. We need all the roles to be played fully in relative reality.

A holistic *Gnana Yoga* practitioner keeps on working while at the same time inquiring deeply into his existence. Two mantras are specifically used in *Gnana Yoga*. One is *So Hum*, which means 'I am that', and *Ahum Brahmasmi*, which means 'I am Brahman'.

TO READ BEFORE AND AFTER MEDITATION

In his book *Dynamic Balanced Living*, Yogi Shanti Desai has compiled a list that reveals the core message of *Gnana Yoga*. It's good to read this list before and after meditation. First you read affirmations of the ultimate reality, then negations of the relative reality.

Affirmations

I AM THE SELF (*ATMAN*)
Spark of God as *Sat*, *Chit* and *Anand*
I AM THE BLISS CONSCIOUSNESS
Uninvolved passive witness to the drama of life
I AM IMMORTAL
Never born, never dying, I am sustained
by the divine energy
I AM PERFECT AND FREE, HERE AND NOW
Nothing or nobody binds me

Negations

I have no race or nationality.
Human race is my nationality.
I have no religion.
Dharma is my universal religion.
I adhere to no dogma or beliefs.

The divine removes my ignorance.

I have no family.

All living creatures are my family members.

I have no home.

The entire universe is my home.

I am without fame or power.

I am a small reflection of the divine.

I own nothing.

Everything is provided by the divine.

I possess no one.

I am here to serve others.

I control nothing.

I am only an instrument. Cosmic laws govern.

I rely on nothing and no one.

Only divine grace and *satsang*.

I am not the intellect.

I rely on divine guidance and intuition.

I am not my emotions.

They change constantly.

I am free from duality.

Free from pleasure-pain, honor-insult.

I am not the mind.

Mind does not exist, it is changing waves.

I am not the senses.

They are only means of perceptions.

I am not the body.

It is vibrating energy and changes constantly.
I am not male or female.
I am spirit without boundaries.
I am not father, son, mother, or sister.
These are roles I play.
I have no name.
Name is just a label.

The term "*I*" in these affirmations and negations always relates to the ultimate reality, *Atman* or pure spirit, not the temporary personality or roles we play. To really grasp the depth and meaning of these statements one must read them often and contemplate them deeply.

Be ever mindful of the fact that these statements merely *point the way*. The state of enlightenment is beyond words and concepts. Food will not satisfy when you only look at it and talk about it. For food to satisfy it must be eaten. The same goes for spiritual truths. It's not enough to read about them and talk about them. Yoga is an active practice. Yoga is a lifestyle.

KARMA YOGA

The word *Karma* means action. For every action there is a reaction. *Karma Yoga* has often been called the yoga of cause and effect, or, the yoga of sowing and reaping, but it is really the *yoga of action*. The goal of the *Karma Yoga* practitioner is to be active and yet remain free from the results of his actions. He serenely accepts the effects of his previous actions and devotes his current actions to service.

Swami Vivekananda had a supreme understanding of *Karma Yoga*. He told his students to work relentlessly and yet not to be attached to their work, so that the mind could remain free. He explained that poverty, riches and happiness, are all *fleeting* and *temporary*; that they are not our essential nature, which is not disturbed by misery or success. According to Vivekananda, *Karma Yoga* is a way of achieving freedom through selflessness and good deeds.

The *Karma Yoga* practitioner need not believe in God, ask piercing questions about the nature of the spirit, or think about philosophical or existential concepts. The *Karma Yoga* practitioner has a job to do and he should simply fulfill that job without attachment to the outcome.

In his books Vivekananda poses questions about the good we can do in the world. He says that because of the fleeting and ever changing nature of the world we can never do permanent good or induce permanent change. The *Karma Yoga* practitioner should simply work for the sake of work, perform good deeds and selflessly serve, even though the fruits of his work may be temporary. *Karma Yoga* is an attitude towards life.

Buddha was a true *Karma Yoga* practitioner and said it aptly: "I do not care to know your various theories about God. What is the use of discussing all the subtle doctrines about the soul? Do good and be good. And this will take you to freedom and to whatever truth there is."

DIFFERENT KINDS OF REACTION

According the *karma* ideology the world is in perfect equilibrium. Energy that is taken from one place will resurface in another. All actions produce reactions and all effects have causes. According to yoga philosophy there are *four kinds* of actions that produce different kinds of reactions.

Sanchita Karma – A collection of effects from previous lives and from the subconscious mind.

Prarabdha Karma – Also known as fate or destiny. The collective reactions or effects of previous actions surface in current life. According to yoga philosophy, this explains why some people are 'lucky' and other can be 'unlucky' and why little children can show signs of very strong character impressions early in life.

Kriyamana Karma – Present actions driven by will and desire. People affect their own future with current actions.

Agami Karma – Instant reactions related to current actions, for example when a person touches a hot stove and gets burned or goes through a tense period and gets a headache.

This concept that everything in the world is in a state of equilibrium and moves to restore balance does not only presuppose that we reap as we sow in this life, but also assumes the existence of *reincarnation*. Even though most religions and philosophies make room for some kind of afterlife, the concept of reincarnation is often met with skepticism and rightly so. There is little evidence to support the claim.

KARMA YOGA AND REINCARNATION

Being very practical and earthbound, I cannot say with any certainty that I believe in reincarnation, but at the same time it is a fascinating philosophy. I must point out that people can practice all aspects of yoga without believing in reincarnation. Yogi Shanti Desai has explained to me many times that the concept is highly theoretical and cannot be proved or disproved, but in his book *Yoga Holistic Practice Manual* he lists **nine reasons** for why it can be beneficial to understand, and even believe in, reincarnation.

1. *We are never too old to attempt something new as age is no barrier, because life is continuous. We learn new spiritual lessons and grow in wisdom as we grow older.*

2. *No spiritual effort is ever wasted. Lord Krishna teaches that devotees on the spiritual path are reincarnated into a pious family and a spiritual environment. They inherit good health, have a zeal for spiritual enlightenment, and continue their spiritual journey.*

3. *We can realize that we are responsible for everything in our life and have created our present situation. We can stop blaming our parents, society, and various situations for our problems. This realization gives deep relaxation. We also can forgive ourselves for making mistakes in the past because we realize that those mistakes were learning experiences.*

4. *As we become responsible we can take charge of our life and improve its quality. We stop hoping for someone else to help us and we don't expect miracles. Instead, we realize that we can create our own miracles. For exam-*

ple, people who want to lose weight or stop smoking are successful only when they decide to take charge of their own life. No self-improvement program will help until one takes charge and assumes responsibility for its success.

5. *Belief in reincarnation removes the fear of death as we consider death to be part of our total life. It can be thought of as a long night for the soul to rest. Like night and day, death and life cycles go on naturally. There is no fear.*

6. *It gives us understanding that there is no escape. Drugs, alcohol, etc. allow you to hide from the fact of life only temporarily. Suicide is not an escape as life will not end nor will it improve until we improve it ourselves.*

7. *We learn to be aware of our thoughts, words, and deeds because we realize that with each thought we are producing karma – positive or negative. We should channel our thoughts in a positive direction, avoiding negative thought patterns. These thoughts will become reality in time. We should learn to perform good deeds without becoming discouraged because no one can take away our reward. What we earn will come to us, and we should prevent producing bad karma because we*

cannot escape punishment for them.

8. *We also learn to escape karma by reducing our mental attachments. By letting go of the feeling of doership and working as an instrument of God, we don't register karma in the memory of our biocomputer. As one evolves, reincarnation is experienced as a conviction. The realization comes to us that the world is in perfect balance and completely systematic.*

9. *Reincarnation increases our love and tolerance for others. Each soul is at a different level of evolution and we should not expect others to be any different. We should remember that we have gone through such experiences ourselves to come to our present level of understanding. It is normal for kindergarten children to learn the alphabet, second graders to read, and high school students to write essays. The world is a school and we are students in different grades learning different lessons. We learn to see the spark of God in everyone in spite of the different human masks they are wearing.*

SWA-DHARMA = PERSONAL PATH

Karma Yoga may appear illusive and unclear at first, but Sri Yogi Hari says it is the foundation for all other paths of yoga. Within *Karma Yoga* the concept of *Dharma* is used to portray a life in harmony with nature and the surrounding universe. Furthermore, the concept of *swa-dharma* is used to portray a personal path each person has chosen in life. According to yoga philosophy we should live in harmony with our *swa-dharma*. Each and every person is special, has talents and creative capacities in a combination that no one else has. There is no need for imitation.

Keep in mind that all actions produce reactions. Sitting around doing nothing is an action in itself and can have both good and bad consequences. The attitude is what matters most. A person can cut another person with a knife for two reasons. One is meant to kill, the other meant to save through a surgical operation. The action, cutting with a knife, is the same, the purposes very different. The *Karma Yoga* practitioner strives to be a force for good, an instrument of love and light.

BHAKTI YOGA

The word *Bhakti* means devotion. *Bhakti Yoga* is the practice of devotion directed towards a higher power. *Bhakti Yoga* is based on human emotions and is often referred to as the yoga of love. The practitioner recites prayers, meditates and devotes his life to God as he understands God. With the practice of *Bhakti Yoga* the line between religion and yoga is blurred considerably, but *Bhakti Yoga* is focused on personal practice and devotion, whereas organized religion has many other purposes and is often involved in political conflicts and other practices that can hardly pass for spiritual practice. *Bhakti Yoga* makes no distinction between religions. It doesn't matter how the practitioner defines his higher power, as long as he cultivates the relationship through prayer and meditation. This kind of tolerance is very relevant.

VIVEKANANDA ON 9/11/1893

For reference I want to share a short speech that Swami Vivekananda made at the world parliament of religions in Chicago on September 11 in 1893.

Sisters and Brothers of America,

It fills my heart with unspeakable joy to rise in response to the warm and cordial welcome which you have given us. I thank you in the name of the most ancient order of monks in the world; I thank you in the name of the mother of religions; I thank you in the name of millions and millions of Hindu people of all classes and sects.

My thanks, also, to some of the speakers on this platform who, referring to the delegates from Orient, have told you that these men from far-off nations may well claim the honor of bearing to different lands the idea of toleration. I am proud to belong to a religion which has taught the world both tolerance and universal acceptance. We believe not only in universal toleration, but we accept all religions as true. I am proud to belong to a nation which has sheltered the persecuted and the refugees of all religions and nations of the earth. I am proud to tell you that we have gathered in our bosom the purest remnant of the Israelites, who came to Southern India and took refuge with us in the very year in which their holy temple was shattered to pieces by Roman tyranny. I am proud to belong to the religion which has sheltered and is still fostering the remnant of the grand Zoroastrian nation. I will quote to you, brethren, a few lines from a hymn which I remember to have repeated from my earliest boyhood, which is every day repeated by millions of human beings: "As the different streams having their sources in different places all mingle their water in the sea, sources in different tendencies, various though they appear, crooked or straight, all lead to Thee."

The present convention, which is one of the most august assemblies ever held, is in itself a vindication, a declaration to the world of wonderful doctrine preached in the Gita: "Whosoever comes to Me, through whatsoever form, I reach him; all men are struggling through paths which in the end lead to me." Sectarianism, bigotry, and it's horrible descendant, fanaticism, have long possessed this beautiful earth. They have filled the earth with violence, drenched it often with human blood, destroyed civilization and sent whole nations to despair. Had it not been for these horrible demons, human society would be far more advanced than it is now. But their time is come; and I fervently hope that the bell that tolled this morning in honor of this convention may be the death-knell of all fanaticism, of all persecutions with the sword or with the pen, and of all uncharitable feelings between persons wending their way to the same goal."

Even though some progress has been made since Vivekananda delivered his speech, it could just as easily have been delivered yesterday. There is still much work to be done if we want to reach the ideal that Vivekananda describes.

THE MANY FACES OF GOD

Concepts of God are man's attempt to understand the universe and his role in it. If a being that we call God created the universe, that same being is hardly playing favorites on this remote planet called Earth which might as well be a speck of dust in galactic terms. Anyone who has ever tried to wrap their head around galactic sizes knows how hard that is. Trying to understand the maker and sustainer of that universe is even harder.

BRAHMAN

In yoga the concept of a higher power has at least two distinctions. One is the concept of *Brahman*, who is the one without a second, which rhymes very well with modern understanding in physics, which theorizes about a *connective field of consciousness* which underlies the energy field of atoms.

According to yoga philosophy nothing exists but *Brahman*, and so everything is *Brahman*. Nothing and no one can explain *Brahman*. Language is too small a medium, since it too is a part of *Brahman*. And so the spirit, *Atman*, is a part of *Brahman* (like everything else).

If *Brahman* is the ocean, *Atman* is the drop. Knowing the essence of the drop you can know the essence of the ocean.

The yoga practitioner can tap into the essence *Brahman*, by unveiling his core identity, *Atman*.

Scientists that get acquainted with the concept of *Brahman* often become very interested. Ken Wilber gives a variety of examples of that in his book *Quantum Questions* which contains the mystical writings of top tier scientists.

ISHWARA = GOD

In yoga philosophy there is also a concept that has a closer link to modern religious assertions. Since *Brahman* has all qualities, then *Brahman* has no distinctive qualities. From that lack of distinction the concept of *Ishwara* was born. *Ishwara* is similar to the Western concept of God, which has qualities.

As soon as people ascribe any qualities, call out to God, say the he/she/it is good, bad, the creator, is full of love or anything else for that matter, then they are referring to *Ishwara* according to the philosophy of yoga.

The concept of *Ishwara* is in harmony with descriptions of God in all the major religions except Buddhism, which does not ascribe to a concept of God.

POLYTHEISM OR MONOTHEISM

For further distinction, *Ishwara* is divided into three parts, related to birth, life and death. These three qualities or distinctions then appear in mythology as three separate Gods, the creator *Brahma* (not to be confused with *Brahman*), the sustainer *Vishnu* and the destroyer or transformer *Shiva*, sometimes called *Mahesh*.

When *Ishwara* (God with qualities) sends messengers to the people of Earth, they are called *Avatars* (Jesus, Buddha, Krishna, etc.). You see how far removed the concept of *Avatar* has become in our society today through movies and video games, which is one more example of how the overuse of a specific term that is been taken out of context can dilute its meaning.

These kinds of distinctions keep going within yoga philosophy and that is why many people think that both yoga and Hinduism preach *polytheism*. But the concept of *Brahman* is at the core of these distinctions and so these approaches are *monotheistic*.

NADA YOGA

One of form of *Bhakti* or devotion is *Nada Yoga*. The practitioner of *Nada Yoga* uses harmony, rhythm and music to connect to his higher power, God or *Nada Brahman*. At first glance *Nada Yoga* practitioners might look like ordinary musicians, but they are using music as a vehicle for spiritual practice. The first step in *Nada Yoga* is musical ability. You start by learning to play instruments and sing mantras. With increased capability, the music is allowed to take over, and the vibrations will allow you to enter conscious spiritual states of awareness. For further clarity I have decided to include a short chapter from Sri Yogi Hari's book titled *Chants*:

Nada Yoga is the science of using vibration to connect with God, or Brahman, the one without a second, or the all-pervading consciousness. Brahman manifests in this universe as vibration. This first manifestation of the absolute is referred to as OM or Nada Brahman. It is the immutable essence underlying all creation. This is the highest state of divine vibration and is referred to as the Para state. This vibration then becomes differentiated into the primordial elements of sattva, rajas and tamas. These are the gunas, which form the building blocks of all creation. The gunas compose the Pashyanti state, or second level of divine vibration. These first two vibrational states of Para and Pashyanti are of the realm of transcendence and can only be experienced through deep meditation. The third level of differentiated vibration exists in the mental plane in the form of thought; something that can be conceived by the mind. It is referred to as Madyama. The fourth state of vibration is manifest in the external physical world as audible sound, and is referred to as Vaikhari. The music we hear played on instruments or vocal music for example, is of the fourth state and is only the gross manifestation of vibration. Nada Yoga uses the divine music to move from gross differentiated vibrations to subtle vibrations and eventually into the para state, where God is experienced directly as Nadam.

EVERYONE CAN PRAY

Within these distinctions, everyone should be able to find a *devotional aspect* that fits their upbringing and personality. Within *Bhakti Yoga* it doesn't matter if the prayers are directed towards an undefined higher power, God, Jesus, Shiva, Vishnu, Krishna, Buddha, Allah or any other version of *Brahman*, the one without a second. In *Bhakti Yoga* the emphasis is placed on strengthening ones relationship with a higher power through a variety of devotional methods.

Because of the Hindu connection many of the prayers and mantras within *Bhakti Yoga* are directed towards Hindu deities, which are reflections of *Brahman*. Some Western practitioners of yoga welcome these new distinctions, while others conservatively hold on to their current definitions of God. As an example of this it can be noted that Gandhi made an effort to practice a variety of religious pathways before he settled into devotion to *Rama*, using the *Bhagavad-Gita* as his vehicle for spiritual inspiration. Ramakrishna, who was Swami Vivekananda's teacher took this discipline a step further and invested many years of practice in each of the major religions and is said to have reached the state of enlightenment in all of them.

TRUE WORSHIP

What then is true worship? From the standpoint of *Brahman*, it is seeing the spark of the divine in everything, experiencing the interconnectedness of the universe and experiencing the love that binds it all together. The spark of *Brahman*, *Atman*, is within all of us, no matter what we call it. It is within people of all races, nationalities and religions. The yoga practitioner who has perfected the practice of *Bhakti Yoga* is a source of love and compassion, because he sees the divine in everything. He sees the divine spark, the common ground, how everything is interconnected.

But while progressing towards this state, loving emotions can rise and subside. The practitioner must continuously elevate his base emotions towards love and compassion through prayer and meditation before the loving state becomes permanent, and even then he must work on maintaining it.

A Tibetan monk described it this way. One moment he is a source of love and feels the interconnectedness of all life; the next moment he doesn't understand how anyone can love the limited and often irritating human beings he is surrounded with.

It is important for all practitioners of yoga to differentiate between temporary states and permanent traits at the outset of practice. At one moment the yoga practitioner is

61

enveloped in love and compassion in a beautiful ceremony with his teacher and friends; the next moment he is cursing other drivers in traffic. Tolerance towards others and oneself is a vital component in the practice of *Bhakti Yoga*.

CHRISTIAN CONNECTION

Many Western yoga students, which have been raised within Christianity, ask how it is possible to practice *Bhakti Yoga* and remain devoted to Jesus. There is no contradiction between the two. According to yoga philosophy true worship of Jesus would consist of following his teachings. The idea that Jesus died for our sins and the only thing we have to do is believe in Jesus and pray to him on Sundays, keep a cross or picture of Jesus on the wall and then go about business as usual, doesn't really comply with the ideas of *Bhakti Yoga*. The imagery and reminders are fine, but *Bhakti Yoga* focuses on the *personal practice* of prayer and meditation. Plus, using the teachings and life of Jesus as a template for one's own life will have a much bigger transformational effect.

PATH OF LOVE AND COMPASSION

Bhakti Yoga is the path of love. It is the easiest path within yoga because it is based on elevating human emotions. All the practices within *Bhakti Yoga* focus on raising vibrations from the basic animal instincts we all possess, to the divine love and compassion we also have access to.

With that in mind even *atheists* can adhere to some of these principles. They don't have to believe in God or an architect of the universe. They can simply cultivate kindness, gratitude, tolerance and ethical behavior, because that is what *Bhakti Yoga* produces in a nutshell.

RAJA YOGA (ASHTANGA)

Raja means king or emperor. In the cultural context of ancient India, being king or emperor was the highest position an earthly man could hold. *Raja Yoga* is therefore the highest yoga. The practice of *Raja Yoga* is systematic, scientific and effective. The structure of *Raja Yoga* is divided into eight limbs, and that is why it is also called *Ashtanga*, *ash* meaning eight and *tanga* meaning limbs. The eight limbs are:

Yama
Niyama
Asana
Pranayama
Pratyahara
Dharana
Dhyana
Samadhi

The first two limbs, *yama* and *niyama*, are the ethical guidelines of yoga and are designed to help the practitioner live in harmony with nature and control his animal instincts. These two limbs have been likened to the *Ten Commandments* in Christianity. The practice of *yama* and *niyama* creates real freedom for the practitioner, because there is no freedom without discipline.

Let's take the example of a car. The breaks are the discipline that gives us freedom. If we only had the gas pedal the car would simply be a deathtrap. The same is true about the banks of a river. They are the discipline that directs the water. Without the banks there would be no river, only a sluggish quagmire.

The practice of *yama* and *niyama* is a lifetime endeavor. Very few have reached perfection and therefore it may be more effective to strive for progress than perfection. For the practice to take hold one needs perseverance, patience and tolerance towards oneself and others. Progress in this area can result in well-being, integrity and a stronger connection with spirit.

People who are interested in making the practice of *yama* and *niyama* a priority should read the autobiography of Mahatma Gandhi. He cultivated ethical behavior all his life and according to him, he did not reach perfection.

The third limb, *asana*, was originally meant to prepare the body for meditation. *Asana* literally means *steady posture*, but in today's society it has become synonymous with the physical exercises that most people call yoga. In Patanjali's *Yoga Sutras*, which is the original scripture of *Raja*

Yoga, it is said that the body should be still while meditating. The original *asana* is the *lotus* pose, and in it the practitioner sits with his legs crossed, his back is straight and his head, neck and spine are in vertical alignment.

The fourth limb, *pranayama*, is largely based on breathing exercises that allow the practitioner to gain more control over his life energy. The word *prana* means life energy. The second part of the word can either be interpreted as *yama*, which means control, or *ayam*, which means expansion. *Pranayama* is therefore the expansion and control of life energy.

Together these first four limbs comprise the practice of *Hatha Yoga*. *Ha* means sun and *Tha* means moon, representing the masculine and feminine energies, strength and softness, yang and yin. The goal of *Hatha Yoga* is to regulate the energy flow in the body, strengthen it and prepare it for sitting still in meditation, prayer and contemplation. *Hatha Yoga* has also been presented as forceful yoga. Fire is used to heat and strengthen clay. In the same way the practitioner uses *Hatha Yoga* to strengthen and fortify the body. *Hatha Yoga* also includes six cleansing techniques, *shat kriyas* (see glossary). You will learn more about *Hatha Yoga* in the next chapter.

The fifth limb, *pratyahara*, focuses on controlling the senses. Our consciousness is constantly being drawn to the outside world by our senses (sight, hearing, smell, taste and touch). Yoga philosophy likens the senses to five untamed horses that pull man in all different directions. For us to be able to draw our attention and consciousness inward, we must gain control over our senses.

The sixth limb, *dharana*, or concentration is the starting point of meditative practice. When the practitioner lives in harmony with his surroundings and has control over his basic urges (*yama* and *niyama*), when he has balanced the energy flow within the body and can sit still for long periods of time (*asana* and *pranayama*), and when he can easily divert his attention away from his surroundings by controlling his senses (*pratyahara*), he will have a much easier time controlling his awareness through concentration. Sri Yogi Hari says that an unbroken stream of concentration for two minutes automatically leads one into a meditative state, which is the seventh limb.

The seventh limb, *dhyana*, or meditation, is not an action or practice, but a *state* that the practitioner enters into once he has made all the right preparations. In that respect meditation is much like sleep. It is not something we do, but rather a state we enter into. There are several different methods used to enter the state of meditation, but if practiced diligently they all lead to the same state.

Meditation becomes much less intimidating when people realize that they only have to concentrate in an unbroken stream for two minutes to enter this fourth state of consciousness (*the other states of consciousness being waking, dreaming and deep sleep*).

According to Sri Yogi Hari one enters into the state of *samadhi*, or enlightenment (which is the eight limb), when the state of *dhyana*, or meditation, has been maintained uninterrupted for twenty to thirty minutes (*for the record it must be noted that the times that Sri Yogi Hari gives are not absolute, only good indicators*).

In order to achieve permanent enlightenment, one must enter the state of *samadhi* repeatedly. Similar to stretching a muscle, one must stretch more than once or twice to achieve permanent flexibility. Meditation must be entered into repeatedly on a regular basis to achieve a permanent state of realization or enlightenment.

When *dharana*, concentration, *dhyana*, meditation, and *samadhi*, enlightenment, all occur at the same time (which only happens in the cases of seasoned practitioners), it is called *samyama*.

Everyone can begin to use practices linked to the first six limbs, but since *dhyana* and *samadhi* are states of being, not actions, they cannot be trained specifically. All the practitioner can do is to create the right circumstances and then enter into the states if they present themselves.

In that way there is a strong link between sleeping and meditation. Sleep is a state. If you create the right circumstances you will fall asleep. And yet you don't argue with your friends about which method of falling asleep is the best. If you fall asleep, then your method works. The same is true for meditation. There is not one right way, but there are certainly wrong ways. A person that has trouble falling asleep can probably benefit from learning from a person that falls asleep easily. The same is true with meditation. It's always good to learn from a seasoned practitioner.

When choosing a meditation practice it is wise to choose a practice that has stood the test of time and produced enlightened masters who have passed their knowledge and experience to the next generation. That is how the yoga tradition has been preserved for thousands of years.

DELVING DEEPER

Since *Raja Yoga* is the highest yoga and includes the most number of yogic practices, it is appropriate to delve deeper into each of the eight limbs.

1. YAMA (SELF-CONTROL)

The first five of the ten ethical guidelines focus on *self-control*. If you examine a human fetus when it is growing, it shows striking similarities with a variety of other animal species at different stages, which supports the theory of evolution. While having animal instincts is not all bad (since tendencies of self-preservation, sexual aggression and asserting positions of power have served mankind for centuries) we must admit that these instincts have also caused tremendous pain and disharmony among men. If a person is to grow beyond the animal instincts, she must learn to control the instincts, so she may live in harmony with herself and her surroundings. The practice of yoga increases life energy and personal power and that in turn demands more responsibility and adherence to ethical guidelines.

Ahimsa (non-violence) – A yoga practitioner should not kill or harm another human being unnecessarily or for pleasure. In a wider context *ahimsa* unveils the interconnectedness of all life. Thus the yoga practitioner should avoid harming all together; start at the material level by not harming physically, then learn to control his words, and finally, marinate his thoughts in non-violence. Through awareness and compassion, negativity and hatred can be transformed into love.

Satya (truthfulness) – The yoga practitioner should be truthful and honest in all his actions. To refrain from lying is the traditional practice of *satya*, but exaggerating and gossiping are also forms of lying. For the practitioner to be truthful there must be harmony between thoughts, words and actions. When the practitioner thinks, talks and acts with integrity he unleashes tremendous power. If he thinks one thing, says another and then acts in a third way, then not only is he causing himself unrest, but his power will dwindle and his actions fail.

According to yoga philosophy truth has three measuring sticks: It should be true (*satyam*), good for all (*shivam*) and promote beauty and happiness (*sundaram*).

Asteya (non-stealing) – The average citizen does not steal in the literal sense, and neither does the average yoga practitioner. But on a more subtle level there are other ways of stealing, such as getting awarded without merit or not working wholeheartedly for one's salary.

Brahmacharya (harnessing sexual energy) – *Brahman* means God or absolute reality, *charya* means devotion, but *brahmacharya* is traditionally translated as abstinence from sex or as chastity. Sexual energy is one of the animal instincts that sustain mankind. People spend a tremendous amount of energy trying to fulfill their sexual desires. This focuses awareness and attention away from spiritual practices and into the material world. By harnessing sexual energy the yoga practitioner is able to draw his attention inward, which is both the goal and practice of yoga. The less attention and energy that is given to pleasurable sensations, the more the practitioner can focus on the causal body, the spirit or *Atman*, the drop in the cosmic ocean, known as *Brahman*. By focusing inward the yoga practitioner is showing devotion to *Brahman*, and that is *brahmacharya*.

Harnessing sexual energy is a process of transformation, not repression. If a yoga practitioner tries to repress or contain sexual energy without understanding, it will result in mental and sometimes physical problems. If he abstains because he has been told to or is threatened punishment (*especially punishment from God*), then the discipline is either not likely to last or in the case of some catholic priests and quite a few yogis, the sexual energy may rear its ugly head in very damaging ways.

The yoga practitioner must decide to follow this path of restriction based on *understanding* and know that with practice he may transform the sexual energy into spiritual energy. Understanding must precede the discipline. Then it will produce freedom.

I freely admit that the idea of abstention from sex has not been greeted with open arms by my students through the years. I have pointed out that a form of *brahmacharya* can be attained through the practice of *tantra*, which is a method of using the sexual energy in a loving context for spiritual purposes. The philosophy of *tantra* also unveils a very real difference between men and women, and it must be admitted that most of the yogic texts have been written by men for men, and that the masculine libido tends to be more active and cause more problems. The family oriented yoga practitioner can continue his sexual practices in a loving relationship, bringing more awareness and understanding to sexual acts, and still practice partial *brahmacharya*, harnessing and directing the sexual energy in another fashion.

In a wider context, *brahmacharya* is about harnessing *all life energy* and directing it towards *Brahman*.

Aparigrahah (non-greediness) – This fifth guideline in the self-control category reminds the yoga practitioner not to become greedy or possessive. Relatively little is needed to survive. Acquiring material possessions requires a tremendous amount of energy, much of which could be spent on spiritual practice or selfless service.

2. NIYAMA (POSITIVE ATTRIBUTES)

The second half of the ethical guidelines is about cultivating positive attributes. It is the opposite side of the coin. The guidelines of *yama* focus on controlling existing tendencies, the guidelines of *niyama* are about the cultivation of new and positive attributes.

Saucha (purity) – According to yoga philosophy we are a reflection of the divine. Body, mind and emotions are the vehicles of spirit in this world. The yoga practitioner should make an effort to keep these vehicles or pathways clean. The body is kept clean with physical exercise and a *satvik* (pure) diet, breathing exercises and cleansing. The mind and emotions are cleansed through prayer, *satsang* (positive association), meditation, mantra chanting, and the cultivation of *vairagya* or non-attachment.

Santosa (contentment) – The yoga practitioner who is content possesses a kind of serenity that is essential for his spiritual growth. He is quietly happy and satisfied, non-judgmental and at peace with himself.

Tapas (self-discipline) – Discipline is necessary for everyone that wants to succeed in life, especially those who want to gain self-control. The word *tapas* means heat or heating. For metal to harden it is heated and cooled alternatingly. The same is done with objects made of clay. Discipline builds will and spiritual energy. Self-discipline is based on doing what one sets out to do, *whether one feels like it or not.* Yoga practitioners use self-discipline to adhere to practices and reduce their contact with possibly addictive sensory pleasures, all in an effort to gain more control over their attention.

Self-discipline should never be a form of puritanical self-punishment and should always be done with sufficient

understanding of what the discipline is meant to achieve. The yoga practitioner should therefore always ask: "What is the desired outcome I am aiming for by practicing this form of self-discipline?"

Swadhyaya (introspection and self-study) – The title of this book is related to this guideline. *Know thyself!* Without introspection and self-study one cannot know one's self. The yoga practitioner studies his body, emotions and mind. He looks for the roots of all behavior and thoughts, tries to understand what drives him and why. Everyone changes over time, whether they want to or not. Change can happen reactively or be pursued actively. The yoga practitioner chooses how he would like to change and then behaves accordingly, making adjustments along the way in line with what he finds to be true. Often the changes are minor and take a short time; other times he is unable to change and must simply surrender to that fact, thusly changing his attitude.

Self-study and introspection allow the yoga practitioner to monitor changes, to see whether he is progressing or regressing, so that he may make the necessary changes. Over time self-study produces non-attachment. With the inevitable changes one goes through, it becomes easier to see the body and personality as transitory, and attach ones identity to the unchanging reality of *Atman*.

Ishwara Pranidhana (surrendering to the divine) – This practice is crystalized in the words *"Thy will be done"*. Through surrender the yoga practitioner becomes a spiritual instrument and allows the divine energy to flow through him. Being still and vibrating at the frequency of the causal body, one attunes to spirit and is open to the will of the divine.

3. ASANA (POSTURE)

Asana means steady posture. The original posture taught within the confines of *Raja Yoga* was the *lotus* pose, in which the practitioner sits with his legs crossed and his spine, neck and head are vertically aligned. The *lotus* pose is stable and it reduces blood flow to the legs, which increases blood flow to other areas of the body, including the spine and brain which are the main instruments used in meditation.

In order to progress and include the following five limbs in this eight limbed system it is important to be able to *calm down the body and keep it in a stable posture for a prolonged time*. For beginners this steady pose can be assumed sitting on a chair. Stiff hips are common in the West and the *lotus* pose is out of reach for many, but being able to sit still is imperative if one is to progress. Other physical postures have surfaced over the years and with the branding and trademarking of yoga in modern society they have multiplied exponentially. Yoga postures will be dealt with in more detail in the chapter on *Hatha Yoga*.

4. PRANAYAMA (ENERGY CONTROL)

The word *prana* means life energy and the second part of the word *prana-yama* is said to mean either *yama*, which means control, or *ayam*, which means expansion. *Pranayama* is therefore the control and expansion of life energy.

The practice of *pranayama* is mostly based on breathing exercises. The breath and *prana* are closely intertwined. In yogic texts it is said that control of breath leads to control of the life energy. Yogis have in many cases achieved such a degree of control over their bodily functions through concentration and breath control that they can effectively manipulate their body temperature and affect their heart rate.

While being open to those possibilities, the goal of the average practitioner should be much more mundane to begin with. Increased control of breathing usually increases *energy* and *stabilizes emotions*. The energy increase is connected with increased oxygen flow and the emotional stabilization is due to the link between breath and emotion. When people become emotionally unstable, i.e. fearful, anxious, angry or irritated, their breathing usually becomes shallow, fast and irregular. When their emotions are stable, breathing is usually deep, steady and regular. In order for

78

the yoga practitioner to be able to enter into a state of deep meditation, breath control is extremely important.

Yoga offers a variety of breathing practices. The three most important ones are deep abdominal breathing, cleansing breath or *kapalabhati,* and alternate nostril breathing or *anuloma viloma.* You can look these up on the web if you want to learn them, but as with everything, it is much better to learn them directly from an experienced teacher if possible.

5. PRATYAHARA (SENSE CONTROL)

The five senses (touch, sight, smell, taste and hearing) navigate man's existence and help him to survive and thrive in the external world. But when the yoga practitioner decides to turn his attention inward, the senses become an obstacle. The practitioner has a few possible options. One is to manipulate his surroundings in such a way that he is not disturbed. He does this by closing his eyes, stimulates neither the senses of taste or smell, reduces environmental sounds or drowns them out with soft sounding music, and makes sure that his clothing is comfortable and that he is neither too hot or too cold.

People often ask about the use of incense in this context. The original purpose of incense was to mask other assailing smells. In the ancient East there was no air conditioning, plumbing or waste disposal, so that odors of food, sweat and feces, to name a few, were often in the air close to where yoga was being practiced. In those circumstances the use of incense made sense. Now, their use is mostly symbolic and can actually cause a disturbance in the mind by over stimulating the sense of smell.

The yoga practitioner cannot always control his surroundings. That is why he trains his senses and increases his control over them so that he may withdraw his attention from the senses when he so desires. This is called *becoming the tortoise.*

Numbing the senses is not the same as training them. A person that is under the influence of alcohol or drugs often withdraws his attention from the senses because they have been numbed. But the use of such aids never leads to permanent enlightenment, although many people say they have had temporary spiritual experiences while under the influence.

The yoga practitioner chooses a more time consuming but less costly way of training his senses, so that he may overcome heat, cold, smells and sounds.

Training the senses is a difficult process and therefore the beginner needs to control his environment as much as possible. But if a seasoned practitioner of yoga cannot practice in more difficult circumstances without letting the environment disturb him, then he has not progressed in the practice of *pratyahara.*

6. DHARANA (CONCENTRATION)

Nothing significant can be achieved without concentration. Whether it is in the area of self-control, work, study, sports or relationships, concentration is always beneficial. In *Raja Yoga* the practitioner practices maintaining his concentration on one object. Concentration can be likened to harnessing the rays of the sun through a magnifying glass. Scattered the rays of the sun are not powerful, but when gathered and concentrated on one object they can start a fire.

The yoga practitioner increases his concentration abilities by focusing on something that under normal circumstances does not require a lot of concentration, for example the act of sitting still and following the breath. Short *mantras* and prayers can also become the objects of concentration in yoga.

A parable tells of a young student who was rewarded by his teacher for the progress he had made on the spiritual path. The teacher said the student could have anything he wished for. The student asked for a *magic genie* that the teacher possessed, so that he could have all his wishes fulfilled. The teacher warned him that the genie needed to be constantly active or else he would destroy his owner. The student was self-assured and said that he wouldn't be running out of wishes any time soon. But two days later the student returned, frightened, unrested and anxious. He told his teacher that as soon as he got home he had wished for a palace and thought that might keep the genie occupied for a while, at least for a couple of days, but the wish was fulfilled within minutes. Mindful of the warning his teacher had given him, the student scrambled to find another wish, and then another, and another. The genie fulfilled them one by one. Pretty soon the student had run out of wishes and now he was hiding from the genie so that he would not be destroyed. He begged is teacher to help him. The teacher knew something like this would happen and had a solution ready. He told the student to have the genie build a high tower and then tell the genie to go up and down the tower continuously until the next time he was needed. Thusly the student got the genie under control and could enjoy its powers.

As with all good parables this story can be interpreted in a variety of different ways. The imagery can for example easily be transferred onto the mind. The mind is the genie that can fulfill all our wishes, but at the same time it can destroy us little by little if left to its own devices. A mind that is out of control can induce stress, anxiety, fear, tension, anger, jealousy, irritation and the list could go on and on. The tower in the story can be seen as any method of concentration that will keep the mind busy when it is not in use, such as focusing on the breath or repeating a mantra.

And so, when the mind is not being used, the yoga practitioner directs it towards a practice that keeps his mind anchored. He focuses on the breath, a mantra, or a prayer, instead of allowing the mind to become restless. With practice, both passively sitting and actively focusing on the breath during the day, the yoga practitioner increases his concentration to a point that will eventually lead him into a state of meditation.

7. DHYANA (MEDITATION)

According to Sri Yogi Hari the mind automatically falls into a state of meditation when a stream of concentration is unbroken for two minutes or longer. Meditation is sometimes called *turyia* or the fourth state. It can be likened to a *wakeful deep dreamless sleep*, because it is neither waking, nor dreaming, nor deep dreamless sleep, and actually produces a different set of brainwaves than the other three states. It is a state of wakefulness that is void of the dreaming state (often referred to as the restless mind). In this state, pure consciousness is unveiled. It is sometimes called the silent witness, because it witnesses our thinking processes and our bodily movements.

All Eastern philosophy agrees that pure consciousness is at the core of the human being. Yoga philosophy calls it *Atman*, while others have named it spirit, self, soul, or silent witness. Whichever concept or word people choose, this pure consciousness (still another name) is *beyond* the world of concepts and words, and can hardly be described, merely pointed to.

One way of pointing to pure consciousness is to liken it to *the eye of a storm*. When the storms of the body, emotions and mind seem to be taking over, the practitioner can revert to the eye of the storm through meditation, regain conscious contact with pure consciousness and establish peace of mind.

Many books have been written to glorify differing methods of meditation. But when the practitioner understands that meditation *is a state not a practice*, the type of practice becomes less important and practicing becomes more important. The chosen form of practice simply needs to predictably generate the state of meditation most of the time. Books and teachers can increase the practitioners understanding and give him a frame to work within, but *only through personal practice* can he attain the experience of meditation. Only through persistent and regular practice can the yoga practitioner reveal the *Atman*.

Eloquent descriptions of the state fade in comparison to direct experience. This has been a core problem for spiritual masters through the ages. How can they encourage their students to meditate when they only have words to describe a state that is beyond words and emotions? Their attempts have been likened to describing a rainbow to a person that has been blind from birth. Nothing short of gaining sight can give that person a firsthand experience of what a rainbow looks like. However, when sight is lacking, it's better to get descriptions than nothing. The key difference is that yoga practitioners can certainly reach the meditative state through practice, whereas the blind person is unlikely to gain sight. Meditation practices are easy to learn, but only through regular practice can one attain the meditative state.

8. SAMADHI (SELF-REALIZATION)

According to yoga philosophy there are two types of enlightenment. One is called *sarbij samadhi*, or enlightenment with seeds, closely related to the idea of *Karma Yoga* where each action produces a reaction or seed. When the yoga practitioner reaches *sarbij samadhi* he continues to sow seeds with his actions and has to deal with the consequences in this life or the next. Thus the practitioner is still said to be bound to the cycle of birth and death, even though he is *constantly aware of his pure and unchanging identity*. The supreme goal of yoga according to the scriptures is to be free from this cycle, and when the practitioner enters the state of *nirbij samadhi* that goal has been reached. In the state of *nirbij samadhi* it is like the seeds have been roasted and actions no longer produce further effects. In between *sarbij* and *nirbij samadhi* there are said to be at least seven stages. Some yoga teachers say that real spiritual life doesn't begin until one has reached the state of *sarbij samadhi*.

These ideas about enlightenment are highly theoretical and people who are at the beginning stages of yoga practice often get caught up in them prematurely. Since neither meditation nor enlightenment can be practiced as such, it is much more effective to focus on the practices leading up to these states and to cultivate the attitudes and practices related to *Karma, Bhakti* and *Gnana Yoga* for support.

HATHA YOGA (KUNDALINI)

Hatha Yoga is traditionally defined as a part of *Raja Yoga*. It is comprised of the terms *Ha* (sun) and *Tha* (moon). *Hatha Yoga* is meant to balance the energy flow in the body, igniting the life energy or *prana* through breathing exercises and postures, and eventually lead to the kindling of the *Kundalini* energy which is said to lie dormant at the base of the spine. When *Hatha Yoga* is practiced fully it becomes the real *Kundalini Yoga*. *Hatha Yoga* is comprised of six components: Ethical guidelines (*yama and niyama*), postures (*asana*), breath or energy control/expansion (*pranayama*), energy locks (*bandhas*) and six cleansing techniques (*shat kriyas*).

HEALTH BENEFITS

Hatha Yoga is usually practiced for health reasons and in that form it has gained tremendous popularity in the West. Most people who start to practice simple postures and breathing techniques experience great health benefits. Regular practice has been shown to strengthen the core muscles, reduce tensions in the major muscle groups and sinews, strengthen and stretch the extremities, improve digestion, stimulate the endocrine system, improve hormonal balance, increase blood flow to all areas in the body, decrease discomfort in the joints, increase oxygen flow, and the list can go on. It is no wonder that *Hatha Yoga* has become so popular in the West. With all its health benefits and relaxing qualities, those who have not yet tried it should take the first step and become convinced.

SEVEN CATEGORIES

When practicing *Hatha Yoga* one should be sure to include practices from all the following seven categories to get the major health benefits.

1) *Warm ups and strengthening*, for example sun salutations, plank, Indian pushups, abdominal and back strengthening, warrior pose and other standing postures.

2) *Inverted postures*, for example headstand (advanced), shoulderstand and plough, or other postures that invert the body and increase blood flow to the abdomen, spine and head.

3) *Forward bends*, for example sitting or standing forward bends to stretch the back of the legs, the spine and back, and to massage the internal organs.

4) *Backward bends*, for example the cobra, the bridge, the wheel, the fish, the bow or other similar poses that bend the spine backwards, to stimulate the kidneys, relieve tension in the back, stretch the abdomen, hips, front of legs and neck, stimulate the thyroid and in some cases massage the internal organs.

5) *Spinal twists*, for example sitting, standing or lying down spinal twists to limber up the spine, massage internal organs and stimulate/balance the nervous system.

6) *Meditation poses*, such as the lotus, half lotus, cross legged position or sitting on heels, with the back straight and the head, neck and spine vertically aligned.

7) *Relaxation poses*, such as the corpse pose, to relax the body and assimilate all the benefits of the physical practice.

Any variation of *Hatha Yoga*, no matter how it has been branded, should be comprised of at least one pose from each of these categories and include breathing practices to offer the full benefits of *Hatha Yoga*.

In the creative and competitive atmosphere produced by the popularity of yoga, many people are only teaching a fraction of what might otherwise be called *Hatha Yoga*, such as only warm ups and strengthening poses. The results are usually diluted and based on a shallow understanding of the holistic benefits *Hatha Yoga* can produce if practiced fully.

If you sign up for a yoga class, you are likely to be taught a form of *yoga fitness* that is based on *Hatha Yoga*. Practices that include postures and breathing are always based on *Hatha Yoga*. Names such as *Iyengar*, *Sivananda*, *Bikram*, *Kripalu*, *Astanga*, and *Anusara*, are not different paths of yoga, but trademarks for differentiation, all based on the foundation of *Hatha Yoga* (see glossary for more on the different brands of *Hatha Yoga*).

Many people think that the practice of *Hatha Yoga* should progress to include constantly more difficult poses. This misunderstanding often leads to misguided directions in so called 'advanced' yoga classes. If flexibility were the only thing required for enlightenment, most circus performers would be much more enlightened than those who practice yoga. The incessant focus on strength and flexibility in the West has in fact drawn attention away from the original goal of yoga, which is to draw attention inwards and create harmony between body, mind and spirit. Instead, people become obsessed with their physical abilities and appearance and stunt their spiritual growth.

CONTROLLING LIFE ENERGY

The ultimate goal of *Hatha Yoga* is not limited to health benefits, but focuses on the control and expansion of the life energy or *prana*. According to yoga philosophy the control of *prana* can result in the kindling of *Kundalini* (an intense spiritual energy which generates instant enlightenment according to the scriptures). But, according to Yogi Shanti Desai, the *Kundalini* concept is highly theoretical, while the increased control of *prana* is accessible to all.

The control and expansion of *prana* is gained through breathing (*pranayama*), energy locks (*bandhas*) and controlled postures (*mudras*), which resemble *asanas*, but are held for a longer period of time. These practices require the body to be healthy, strong, flexible, and free from tension and restlessness. Controlling the breath eventually leads to more control over *prana*, which flows through energy channels called *nadis*, a system which is very similar to the nervous system. Yoga philosophy makes a clear distinction between the nerves and *nadis*, maintaining that the 72.000 *nadis* are the nervous system of the astral body. Of the reported 72.000 *nadis*, there are three main energy channels, called *Ida* (feminine current), *Pingala* (masculine current) and *Shushumna*, main energy channel which lies adjacent to the spine. You might be interested to know that the three energy channels form the *international medical sign*, which is a staff (*Shushumna*) enveloped by two snakes (*Ida* and *Pingala*).

Along the pathway of the spine or *Shushumna*, there are said to be situated seven energy wheels or *chakras*, from the tailbone to the crown of the head (see glossary for more on the *chakras*).

The end goal of *Hatha* or *Kundalini Yoga* is to control *prana* or the life energy in such a way that the energy flows evenly through the channels of *Ida* and *Pingala*, thus kindling the *Kundalini* energy at the base of the spine and channeling it up through *Shushumna*, igniting every *chakra* or energy wheel on the way.

The ideology surrounding the *Kundalini* energy is very enticing. However, both my teachers, Yogi Shanti Desai and Sri Yogi Hari, say that they have not completely awakened this energy despite years of practice. On the other hand, both of them have increased control over their life energy or *prana*. That should be the goal of the average yoga practitioner.

It must also be noted that quite a few people walk this Earth claiming to be *Kundalini* masters. However hard their claims are to refute, both my teachers have met a number of these people who claim to have mastered *Kundalini*, and based on conversations, knowledge of scriptures, and their extensive experience, both men say that they have yet to meet a master of *Kundalini*, even though many of these people have gained more control over their life energy. Increased flow of *prana* can in fact induce some unusual sensations, such as heat or intense sensitivity, especially around the spine, that can lead people to erroneously think that they have kindled the *Kundalini* energy.

KUNDALINI WARNINGS

In most of the yoga books I have read, the yoga practitioner is warned against trying to prematurely awaken or kindle the *Kundalini* energy, especially without the guide of an experienced teacher who has already mastered the path (*of which there may be fewer than reported*). The reason is that this energy is said to be extremely powerful and possibly volatile. Minor physical aches and pains and any mental instability (such as obsessions, depression and other mental illness), can increase exponentially if the practitioner prematurely kindles the *Kundalini* energy.

Warnings say that premature kindling can result in severe health problems and even lead to insanity. That is one more reason why it is important to practice physical cleansing (*shat kriyas*) and increase mental resilience by following the ethical guidelines (*yama* and *niyama*).

HATHA YOGA IS SAFE

I can safely say that practicing the postures and breathing exercise related to *Hatha Yoga* have nothing but positive effects, so long as the practitioner doesn't overuse the energy locks (*bandhas*) and controlled postures (*mudras*).

Simple postures (*asanas*) and breathing techniques (*pranayama*) practiced every day can increased the life energy (*prana*) and reduce lethargy, physical pain and tiredness. The main purpose of *Hatha Yoga* for the regular practitioner should be to condition the body to sit still for long periods of time without becoming stiff or restless, thus making the practitioner able to enter the state of meditation. Swami Sivananda said: "Health is the greatest wealth; peace of mind is the greatest blessing. Yoga gives you both."

EPILOGUE ON RAJA/HATHA YOGA

Raja Yoga is a time consuming practice. It is not for everyone and to reach its higher stages it demands a lifetime commitment. However, for those who want to use practices from *Raja Yoga* for their health and overall wellbeing, I want to point out a progression taught to me by Yogi Shanti Desai.

In the beginning the yoga practitioner should focus on taming the body with postures, include a few select breathing practices and practice a short relaxation/meditation.

With time the proportions should change. The physical exercises should take a shorter time and focus on *maintaining* strength and flexibility, while breathing practices should take more time and meditation practices get more attention.

Once fully established in the practice of *Raja Yoga* the practitioner should only do a few physical exercises, focus on the most effective breathing techniques and invest more time in meditation, effectively reversing the proportions from when he started.

Through this approach the practice will inch towards more depth, instead of ever increasing focus on the physical body, which according to yoga philosophy, is only a temporary reflection of the spirit, *Atman*.

REGULAR PRACTICE

Yoga is about prioritizing. You cannot do everything and therefore you must ask: "Which, if any, of the yoga practices will have the most positive effects on my life right now?" There are no right or wrong answers. This is your life and it is your decision.

If you are interested in proceeding, you may want to focus on your inclinations. Are you driven by action (*Karma* and *Raja Yoga*), emotion (*Bhakti Yoga*) or intellect (*Gnana Yoga*)? Once you have uncovered your inclinations you can choose practices accordingly.

TEMPORARY STATES – PERMANENT TRAITS

I want to remind you of the difference between *temporary states* and *permanent traits*. While practicing yoga you will experience pleasurable physical sensations, peace of mind and calmness. But to begin with, these feelings will likely be short lived. The more often you enter into the temporary states through regular practice, the more likely you are to gain permanent access to them and incorporate permanent traits. This may not be a linear journey. Growth can come in bursts. You will go through periods when you take large strides forward and then you will go through periods when you feel you are making no progress. Persist! It is important to be patient and persevere in the lulls of life. In that way you will make your practice an integral part of your life and then your life will become your practice. *Here are some ideas about how you can practice each of the four major paths of yoga.*

RAJA AND HATHA YOGA PRACTICE

In order to fully practice *Raja Yoga* you need ample time and a strong will. Adhering to the ethical guidelines requires a lifetime of practice and understanding so that it doesn't turn into painful repression. The goal is to discipline the mind and body, not to repress both into submission. Forces of nature will not be repressed, only directed.

If you want to practice *Hatha Yoga*, then it is relatively easy to put together a routine of postures (*asanas*) and breathing techniques (*pranayama*). You can get all the major benefits by practicing postures, breathing and relaxation for 30-90 minutes 3-7 times a week. The main goal is to achieve strength and flexibility so you can sit still for long periods of time without becoming stiff or restless.

When Sri Yogi Hari lived with his master Swami Vishnu-Devananda he practiced *Hatha Yoga* for four hours every day, two hours in the morning and two hours in the afternoon. He reaped like he sowed and became a master of *Hatha Yoga*. However, in his trip to Iceland in 2005 he confessed to me that he wished he would have spent more time with his family and less on his physical yoga practice. That was a big lesson for me.

Breathing practices should become the main emphasis of *Hatha Yoga* when you progress. At first you can study *Hatha Yoga* with an experienced teacher, but with time you should engage in *solitary practice* for more depth.

For you to progress in the disciplines of sense control (*pratyahara*), concentration (*dharana*) and meditation (*dhyana*) it is also good to get the guidance of an experienced teacher in the field. Meditative practices can take anywhere between 10-60 minutes a day.

Simplified practice: Practice a 30 minute *Hatha Yoga* routine 3-5 times a week, include postures from every group (see chapter on *Hatha Yoga*), meditate for 10-20 minutes daily and read about one ethical guideline before or after meditation.

KARMA YOGA PRACTICE

The practice of *Karma Yoga* is the cultivation of an attitude, working for the sake of work, without attachment to the reward and providing selfless service.

Simplified practice: Practice sowing positive seeds with your thoughts and actions and provide selfless service whenever you get the chance.

BHAKTI YOGA PRACTICE

Everyone who develops their faith through prayer or meditation is engaged in a form of *Bhakti Yoga*. The same goes for those who practice tolerance and loving kindness. *Bhakti Yoga* ignites positive and loving emotions. It is the easiest path. You can practice prayer, meditation, chanting, communion, giving thanks, or other simple forms of devotion. Having said that I want to remind you of what Vivekananda said when he warned people about "sectarianism, bigotry, and its horrible descendant, fanaticism" in his 1893 speech.

Simplified practice: Pray when you awake and before you go to sleep, give thanks every day, chant, surrender your life to a higher power, and cultivate loving kindness.

GNANA YOGA PRACTICE

The practice of *Gnana Yoga* is essentially peering into the depth of one's own being to gain self-knowledge. It is important to find a teacher to help on this path, which is said to be the most difficult on within yoga.

Simplified practice: Read the affirmations and negations by Yogi Shanti Desai, provided in the chapter about *Gnana Yoga*, before and after meditation.

HOLISTIC OR INTEGRAL PRACTICE

To develop a holistic yoga practice you can do a little bit of everything. This shouldn't take longer than 60 to 70 minutes a day in simplified form, but if you go deep in each discipline, it can consume all your time.

The goal of yoga is to harmonize the connection between body, mind and spirit, while peacefully co-existing with nature and society. To further understand the integral way of thinking I highly recommend a book titled *Integral Spirituality* by one of the great thinkers of our time, Ken Wilber.

DANGERS ON THE SPIRITUAL PATH

Self-centeredness (not on the everlasting Self, but the temporary self) is the main danger when practicing yoga. Humility is the antidote and must be maintained as one evolves on the spiritual path. As soon as someone claims to be a master or *guru*, that same someone has lost his humility and has stopped progressing. The words master or *guru* should only be used by students when applicable. You see, there can be no masters or *gurus* if there are no humble students. Only through humility can the student see the teacher as a master or *guru*. Using the metaphor from earlier in the book, all sides of the pyramid lead to the same point, but self-centered or ego driven personalities can claim that they have reached the top when they are only on the third or fourth step. The following is a *partial list* of other things that can easily go wrong on the spiritual path.

THE DARTH VADER SYNDROME

Biology teaches that the more complex an organism becomes, the more things can go wrong. A single celled organism cannot get cancer, but a more complex organism like a dog can get cancer. The same goes for engineering or computing. The more complex the structure, the more things can go wrong. Ken Wilber has coined a term for this in relation to spiritual practice. He calls it the *Darth Vader Syndrome* (referencing the Star Wars movies by George Lucas). The more a human being advances spiritually, the more things can go wrong. The spiritual aspirant must therefore always remain aware on the spiritual path. Smugness, arrogance, greed, sexual attraction, and a variety of other similar traps can creep up on the aspirant at any point in his practice, if he lets down his guard. And remember, even though a person can be highly advanced in one area of life, for example in her spiritual practice, that same person can be severely unhinged in another, for example in her sexual conduct.

ESCAPISM

Many people have used spiritual practices as an escape route from other areas of life. They flee their family, stop paying bills, and stop being useful citizens in the name of spirituality. This is escapism. The true spiritual aspirant should prosper in all areas of life, including the material, physical, emotional, mental and spiritual areas.

CO-DEPENDENCY

This tendency can be explained with the words "I am not enough". We have all been guilty of acting in a co-dependent way at one time or another in our lives. But the spiritual aspirant must not allow co-dependency to *control* his thoughts and actions. A co-dependent individual views other people as the source of his happiness and unhappiness. He cannot be happy unless other people are happy. He fluctuates uncontrollably with his surroundings and cannot be his own master. Co-dependency either shows itself through submission or an incessant need to control. The co-dependent individual believes that he will feel better if he can only get other people to change. But happiness cannot be found in the world, the only real source of happiness is within. Our environment is constantly changing. It can affect our levels of happiness, but it is not the source.

VANITY

Contradictions on the spiritual path are wonderful. Everything is relative. One of my favorite contradictions is related to the practice of *Hatha Yoga*. Spiritual practice reminds us constantly that the body will eventually die and that we should attach our identity to the part which doesn't die, and yet, we are told to spend time every day on maintaining the body. The danger with excessive *Hatha Yoga* practice is that the yoga practitioner may start to believe that the body can become immortal, or he may start to focus more on his appearance than his spiritual progress. The only way to steer clear of vanity is to remember that the goal of life according to yoga is to identify with our pure essence, *Atman*. We are all drops in the cosmic ocean. The spirit is everlasting, but the body will die. We should remember to use the body, our current vehicle, for spiritual practice and service, and not be bound or attached to the things that will eventually change or transform.

EXTERNAL NORMS

We can't please everyone. A big part of becoming free from co-dependency and external norms is coming to terms with the following realization: *We will not like everyone, not everyone will like us and that is OK.*

Sri Chinmoy once said in a television interview that man should be like a leaf. Instead of trying to please the other leaves on the tree, the leaf focuses inwards and gets all its energy from the branch, the trunk, the roots and the Earth, thusly experiencing the interconnectedness of all the leaves.

The spiritual quest is probably the most arduous journey that man can embark upon. But the spiritual journey can be more profitable than any other endeavor. If you become preoccupied by everyday troubles or allow yourself to be drawn into the rat race without reflection or contentment, you will be led astray.

That is why it is so important to associate with spiritually inclined people and attend retreats and seminars that focus on spiritual growth. We cannot wholly escape the influence of our surroundings. That is why it is important to choose a constructive environment if possible.

ETHICAL DETERIORATION

We can tame our animal instincts by cultivating ethical thoughts and behaviors. If left unchecked, the animal instincts will appear as greed, lust, anger, jealousy, selfishness and struggle for power. If people engage in antisocial behavior, such as stealing, lying, greediness and violence, they strengthen the veils that cover their spirit and attach themselves to the unavoidable suffering in the world. People who lack an ethical foundation have trouble trusting others because they don't trust themselves. The ethical guidelines of *yama* and *niyama* were cultivated for this reason.

LAZINESS

Don't be lazy. If you don't do anything nothing happens. Spiritual growth demands work! You cannot expect to advance without action. In *Samkhya*, an essential part of yoga philosophy, we find three elements at the root of all creation. They are *sattva* (purity), *rajas* (energy) and *tamas* (stagnation). To further understand these elements you can imagine different states of water. *Tamas* is the quagmire or swamp, a state of stagnation, lethargy and deterioration. *Rajas* is the raging river, a state of energy. *Sattva* is the deep peaceful lake, a state of calm and peace. If we want to get out of a state of lethargy (*tamas*) we need to energize ourselves (*rajas*). It is *impossible* to rise from a state of lethargy (*tamas*) and enter a state of calmness (*sattva*), without first going through a state of energy (*rajas*).

LACK OF PATIENCE AND PERSISTENCE

Stamina! By charting a course and then taking deliberate steps everyday towards your goal you will reach it in the end. You must be ready to travel over peaks and through valleys. Spiritual growth has often been likened to taking three steps forward and then two steps backward. Cultivate patience. Trust that you will attain your goal and don't give up when you meet resistance. Progress is inevitable if you keep up your practice. Stumbling is also inevitable. We are human after all. A strong character does not develop in a person that never makes any mistakes, but it does develop in a person that keeps on trying despite her mistakes and learns from them. Lack of patience and persistence can surface in all our lives. In order to keep ourselves from coming to a complete halt we must develop an intense desire for enlightenment and completely understand why we have chosen the spiritual path in life.

IN YOUR HANDS

This book was designed to make yoga more accessible to *you*. I have attempted to clarify the core concepts of yoga philosophy and show you how yoga practitioners can use a variety of practices for their spiritual advancement. In that way yoga is more scientific than religion. In the Bible it says: "Seek and ye will find". The yogi says: "Practice and reap the benefits."

Take time to read the glossary and further deepen your understanding by reading some of the books I recommend.

Know thyself!

Gudjon Bergmann
www.gudjonbergmann.com

APPENDIX 1
SANSKRIT GLOSSARY

This glossary includes simple explanations of *Sanskrit* terms used in or related to the book.

Abhyasa – Constant practice. An essential element in the behavior of a yoga practitioner.

Ahimsa – Non-violence. A part of the ethical guidelines in yoga.

Ahum Brahmasmi – I am *Brahman*.

Anuloma Viloma – Alternate nostril breathing.

Aparigrahah – Non-greediness. A part of the ethical guidelines in yoga.

Asana – Steady posture. Also used to describe the physical postures in *Hatha Yoga*.

Ashtanga – The eight limbed system of *Raja Yoga*.

Asteya – Non-stealing. A part of the ethical guidelines in yoga.

Atman – The individual soul or spirit.

Ayam – Expansion.

Bandha – Energy locks used to control the flow of *prana* in the body.

Moola-bandha – Energy lock by the root of the spine (tense pc muscle)

Uddiyana-bandha – Energy lock by the solar plexus (draw in navel)

Jalandhara-bandha – Energy lock by throat (bring chin to chest)

Bhagavan – God in human form, for example Rama, Krishna, Buddha or Jesus. Another word used for same concept is *Avatar*.

Bhakti Yoga – The yoga of devotion and love. One of the four main paths of yoga.

Brahma – The aspect of the almighty that creates.

Brahmacharya – Harnessing sexual energy. A part of the ethical guidelines in yoga.

Brahman – One without second. All is *Brahman*. Nothing exists but *Brahman*.

Chakra – Energy wheel or energy center:

Sahasrara chakra – The seventh energy wheel.
Located: Slightly above the crown of the head.
Color: Purple/Thousand colors.
Represents: Nirbij Samadhi.
Bija mantra: None.
Element: Shunyata (emptiness).
Part of causal body.

Agnya (ajna) chakra – The sixth energy wheel.
Located: On forehead in between eyebrows.
Color: Indigo blue.
Represents: Sarbij Samdhi.
Bija mantra: Aum (Om).
Element: Mahat (intuition).

Part of astral body.

Vishuddha chakra – The fifth energy wheel.
Located: At the root of the neck.
Color: Blue.
Represents: Consciousness of a higher self.
Bija mantra: Hum.
Element: Ether.
Part of astral body.

Anahat chakra – The fourth energy wheel.
Located: By the center of the chest near the heart.
Color: Green/Pink.
Represents: Divine love.
Bija mantra: Yum.
Element: Air.
Part of astral body.

Manipura chakra – The third energy wheel.
Located: Slightly above the navel – solar plexus.
Color: Yellow.
Represents: Identity and need for power.
Bija mantra: Rum.
Element: Fire.
Part of astral body.

Swadhishthana chakra – The second energy wheel.
Located: Just below the navel.
Color: Orange.

Represents: Sensory pleasure.

Bija mantra: Vum.

Element: Water.

Part of the astral body.

Muladhara chakra – The first energy wheel.

Located: By the tailbone.

Color: Red.

Represents: Mans self-preservation instincts.

Bija mantra: Lum.

Element: Earth.

Part of the material body.

Dharana – Concentration. Part of *Raja Yoga.*

Dhyana – Meditation. Part of *Raja Yoga.*

Gnana Yoga – The yoga of knowledge and discernment. One of the four main paths of yoga. Also written as *Jnana.*

Guru – A person or event that leads the student from darkness (*gu*) to light (*ru*), usually a term for a teacher.

Gunas – The three elements of creation.

    Tamas – Degeneration, stagnation, heaviness.

    Rajas – Motion, energy, restlessness, power.

    Sattva – Purity, peace, calmness, depth.

Hatha Yoga – The yoga of physical and energy mastery (*prana/kundalini*). *Ha* means sun. *Tha* means moon.

Different brands of Hatha Yoga:

Iyengar Yoga – Based on the teachings of BKS Iyengar who was the disciple of Krishnamacharya (www.iengaryoga.org).

Sivananda Yoga – Based on the teachings of Swami Sivananda (www.sivananda.org). My teacher, Sri Yogi Hari, was a disciple of Swami Vishnu-Devananda who built the Sivananda Yoga Centers all over the world and was a direct disciple of Swami Sivananda.

Bikram Yoga – Based on the teachings of the former Indian champion of *Hatha Yoga* named Bikram Choudhury. Also known as Hot Yoga, because it is practiced in a heated room (www.bikramyoga.com).

Kripalu Yoga – Orignally named by Amrit Desai in reference to his teacher and guru Swami Kripalu who was also the guru of his brother, Yogi Shanti Desai, who has been my teacher and mentor for many years. A good explanation of *Kripalu Yoga* can be found in the book *Yoga Holistic Practice Manual* by Yogi Shanti Desai under the heading *Sarangati* (Surrender) *Yoga*. Originally *Kripalu Yoga* was the method of entering a deep meditative state and then allowing *prana* to move the body into dancing, deep meditation or yoga postures. Yogi Amrit Desai (then known as *Gurudev*, an honorary title bestowed on *gurus* in general; another common title for *gurus* is *Guruji*) founded the Kripalu Yoga Center in Massachusetts but was effectively banished from there by his students when a sex scandal unraveled. He now teaches a method of yoga called *Amrit Yoga* or *Yoga Nidra* (*nidra* meaning deep yogic sleep). The type of *Kripalu Yoga* taught today has little to do with the original intent of Swami Kripalu and has become more of a brand or trademark than anything else. Today the Kripalu Yoga Center has become a melting pot of different yoga practices combined with other Eastern and New Age practices (www.kripalu.org).

Ashtanga Yoga – The name is originally a description of the eight limbed *Raja Yoga* path, but was used for branding purposes by Sri K. Pattabhi Jois, a student of Krishnamacharya (who also taught BKS Iyengar) and has been used to describe yoga exercises that flow and link breath and postures (www.ashtanga.com).

Anusara Yoga – A new western approach based on the teachings of John Friend who was a student of BKS Iyengar. Is based on a blend of yoga postures and so called universal principles of alignment (www.anusara.com).

Kundalini Yoga – As stated earlier in this book, *Hatha Yoga* is the original *Kundalini Yoga,* but a practice taught by Yogi Bhajan where fast breathing and movement are intertwined, is also presented under the name *Kundalini Yoga* (www.kundaliniyoga.com).

Notes from the author: As the reader has already surmised, the different names within *Hatha Yoga* are mainly devised to brand and market different teaching methods. Despite this being a normal progression of diversification and marketing, this trend has also diluted the term yoga substantially. There are many more brands of yoga than the ones I have described above, and yet it is likely that more brands will emerge within the next years. That is why it is very important for the discerning student to look at the background of the brands or their teachers to see if the brand is a new invention or simply an adaptation of classical *Hatha Yoga*. Examples of this might be the British *Yoga Boxing* and the Icelandic *Rope Yoga*, both new inventions, and then *Iyengar Yoga* or *Sampoorna Yoga*, which are adaptations of the classical approaches to *Hatha Yoga*.

Ishwara – *Brahman* with qualities, referred to as God.

Ishwara Pranidhana – Surrendering to God. A part of the ethical guidelines in yoga.

Jai Bhagvan! – Literal translation is 'May God within Win'. Used as a greeting to honor *Atman* within.

Kapalabhati – Cleansing breath – literal translation 'Shining Skull'.

Karma Yoga – The yoga of action. One of the four main paths of yoga.

Kundalini – According to yoga philosophy *kundalini* is a form of spiritual energy that lies dormant at the root of the spine, coiled like a snake. Through practice this energy can be released, shooting up *Shushumna*, the main energy channel in the body, thus igniting all the *chakras*.

Mahesh – The aspect of the almighty that destroys or transforms. Also known as *Shiva*.

Maya – The great illusion, the transitory world of material objects, lights and shadows.

Mumuksha – Desire for enlightenment or liberation.

Mudra – A controlled steady posture that manipulates the energy flow within the body.

Nadis – 72.000 energy channels in the astral body.

> *Ida* – One of three major *nadis.*
> Represents feminine energy.
> *Pingala* – One of three major *nadis.*
> Represents masculine energy.
> *Shushumna* – One of the three major *nadis.*
> Main energy channel which lies parallel to the spine.

Neti, Neti – Not this, not that. Relates to a practice in *Gnana Yoga.*

Niyama – The cultivation of positive attributes. A part of the ethical guidelines in yoga.

Nirbij – Without seeds (in relation to *samadhi* or enlightenment).

OM (AUM) – The primal sound, origin of all languages, holy vibration or holy trinity. According to Swami Sivananda in his book *Bliss Divine AUM* is everything. *A* represents the material world. *U* represents the astral world. *M* represents the causal world. All trinities can be found within *AUM*, such as *Brahma-Vishnu-Shiva,* past-present-future, creation-maintenance-transformation, waking-dreaming-deep sleep, father-son-holy ghost, *tamas-rajas-sattva,* body-mind-spirit, *sat-chit-ananda,* material world-astral world-causal world.

Patanjali – Wrote the *Yoga Sutras* which had been handed down man to man. Lived two centuries before Christ.

Prakriti – The material world.

Prana – Life energy.

Pranayama – The control and expansion of life energy.

Pratyahara – Sense withdrawal.

Purusha – Spirit/God/Goddess.

Raja Yoga – The scientific approach to yoga. One of the four main paths of yoga.

Rishis – The ancient seers who developed yoga.

Sampoorna – Full or complete.

Sarbij – With seeds (in relation to *samadhi* or enlightenment).

Satsang – A gathering of truth.

Samadhi – Enlightenment. A direct revelation of *Atman*.

Samskaras – Deep seeded longings, desires, tendencies in the subconscious.

Santosa – Contentment. A part of the ethical guidelines of yoga.

Sat Chit Anand – The qualities of *Atman*. Ultimate truth, knowledge and bliss.

Satya – Truth. A part of the ethical guidelines of yoga.

Saucha – Purity. A part of the ethical guidelines of yoga.

Shiva – The aspect of the almighty that destroys or transforms. Also known as *Mahesh*.

Shat Kriyas (also known as *Shat Karmas*) – Six cleansing techniques (for detailed descriptions consult *Hatha Yoga Practice Manual* by Yogi Shanti Desai or *Asana Pranayama Mudra Bandha* by Swami Satyananda Saraswati).

Dhauti – Cleansing the esophagus and stomach.

Vasti – Cleansing the rectum, small intestines and colon.

Neti – Cleansing the nasal passages.

Nauli – Massaging the internal organs with the abdominal muscles.

Trataka – Cleansing the eyes.

Kapalbhati – Cleansing the lungs. Also a breathing practice.

So Hum – I am that. Mantra.

Sharir – Veils or bodies. What is veiling the spirit or soul. Scriptures say: "Lift the veil and see God everywhere."

   Sthoola sharir – Material veil or body.

   Sukshma sharir – Astral veil or body.

   Karan sharir – Causal veil or body.

Swadhyaya – Introspection and self-study. A part of the ethical guidelines of yoga.

Tapas – Self-discipline. A part of the ethical guidelines of yoga.

Turiya – The fourth sate (the other three being waking, dreaming and deep sleep).

Vishnu – The aspect of the almighty that sustains creation.

Viveka – Discernment.

Vairagya – Non-attachment.

Yama – Control.

APPENDIX 2
RECOMMENDED READING

Yoga Holistic Practice Manual – Yogi Shanti Desai

Sampoorna Yoga – Sri Yogi Hari

How to Know God: The Yoga Sutras of Patanjali – Swami Prabhavananda and Christopher Isherwood

The Upanishads – Eknath Easwaran

Bhagavad-Gita: The Song of God - Swami Prabhavananda and Christopher Isherwood

Srimad Bhagavatam: The Wisdom of God - Swami Prabhavananda

Asana Pranayama Mudra Bandha – Swami Satyananda Saraswati

APPENDIX 3 – BIBLIOGRAPHY

Previous books by Gudjon Bergmann.

Yes! You Can Manage Stress (2011)

This book is a must have for anyone who has ever struggled with stress. Following the advice in this book will save you time, money, headaches and heartaches. This book debunks common stress myths, gives the reader a comprehensive understanding of stress and offers five effective stress management habits that will positively enhance life.

Motivation & Peace of Mind (2011)

Quotes from Gudjon's previous books about yoga, self-help, motivation, philosophy, spirituality, smoking cessation and more, including a children's book. Whether you are looking for motivation, peace of mind or both, you will be inspired by reading this book.

Quit Smoking and Be Free! (2011)

Based on his successful smoking cessation seminars and his own experience, Gudjon wrote this short, simple and easy-to-follow book, detailing seven simple steps to a smoke-free life.

The book deals with the preparation, nicotine withdrawal and mind-over-matter methods needed to create a life without tobacco.

Gudjon dedicated ten years of his life to running effective smoking cessation seminars in his native country of Iceland where he helped thousands of people to quit smoking. He has also lectured extensively on tobacco prevention for youth and cancer groups.

Balance: The Seven Human Needs Simplified (2011)

This book gives simple guidance about balancing seven important human needs. Based on his 2006 work, 'The Seven Human Needs', Gudjon has compiled this simplified guidebook that gets straight to the point and more user friendly than the original version.

Gudjon bases his need analysis on the ancient Indian *chakra* system, but has solidified his approach through the years through comparisons with the works of Abraham Maslow, Howard Gardner, Tony Robbins, Plato and Ken Wilber, to name a few. From a vast philosophical background springs a simple idea about balance.

Each need is explained in a chapter that includes a contemplation, practical advice, examples of imbalance and positive affirmations.

Create a Safe Space (2011)

This valuable guidebook is intended for yoga teachers. In the book Gudjon shares his experience. He is an experienced yoga teacher (E-RYT 500), ran his own studio from 2001 to 2006, has taught well over 6000 yoga classes, has written seven books based on yoga, and has trained 80 yoga teachers.

Topics include clear boundaries between teachers and students, personal practice, teaching philosophy, time management, self-confidence, the myth of the yoga voice, marketing, boredom, using prior experience, encouraging growth and questioning, ethics and more, all the time drawing on the author's years of experience and his interactions with his yoga teacher trainees through the years.

The book is not written for any specific style, branch or brand of yoga, but for all yoga teachers, regardless of their affiliations and background.

Experienced yoga teachers may find this book helpful for comparing ideas and approaches, the book may even appeal to teachers in general, because of its emphasis on the student-teacher relationship and practical applications.

Living in the Spirit of Yoga (2010)

A 'how to' yoga book for the 21st Century that includes twenty four topics and over 70 practices for mind, body and spirit. Topics include prioritizing daily life, breathing, concentration, taming the senses, discernment, self-discipline, developing a steady posture, meditation, love, non-attachment, letting go of the past, understanding cyclical energy and the energy centers, the importance of self-knowledge and more.

Some of the 70 practices have been simplified based on ancient yogic approaches. From this book you can learn classic postures and breathing techniques plus relaxation and meditation practices. In addition there are practices that focus on expanding love, creating peer groups focused on self-development, flowing, surrendering and accepting life, staying steadfast while developing self-discipline, developing increased self-awareness and self-knowledge, and much more.

This book is truly applicable to the 21st Century. It is free of dogma and absolutes. It invites the reader to pick and choose from a buffet of ideas and practices. But, while the author has tailored the yogic philosophies and practices to modern life he has also stayed true to the core yogic ideas of self-knowledge and self-mastery, true to the heart of yogic empathy and universal love, and true to actions of service.

This book can complement a regular yoga practice and is a must read for everyone interested in a spiritual practice and better quality of life.

The Seven Human Needs (2006)

This book presents a compilation of ideas from broad spectrum. Using the Indian chakra system as a foundation, Gudjon has infused together ideas from Plato, Maslow, Gardner, Wilber and Robbins. The premise of the book is that we are all looking for balance and that the sometimes contradicting human needs can both help us and hinder in our attempt to create a balanced life.

Each need is explained in a chapter that includes a contemplation, practical advice, examples of imbalance and positive affirmations.

The book also provides chapters about how we can live in harmony, how we can apply the model of the seven human needs to everything from politics, to marketing, to relationships. There are also chapters about personal growth and ways to cultivate a personal practice based on this model.

Books in Icelandic - Out of Print

Before Gudjon Bergmann started writing in English he wrote eight books in Icelandic, including two books about yoga exercises, one book about the chakra system, two self-development books, one yoga philosophy book, a children's book and a book about smoking cessation. Combined these books sold 26.000 copies but are currently out of print.

www.ingramcontent.com/pod-product-compliance
Lightning Source LLC
Chambersburg PA
CBHW070148290526
45789CB00002B/684